The Manhattan Diaries Series

# Urban Elixir
## NYC's Proven Blueprint
## To Timeless Skin

Manhattan Allure
Just Like That

# The Manhattan Diaries Series

## Manhattan Allure ~ Just Like That

## Manhattan Vitality ~ Just Like That

## Manhattan Lifestyle ~ Just Like That

## Manhattan Ambition ~ Just Like That

The Manhattan Diaries Series

# Urban Elixir
# NYC's Proven Blueprint
# To Timeless Skin

Manhattan Allure
Just Like That

JESSICA BROOKS

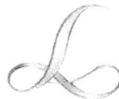

Urban Chronicles Publishing House
an imprint of The Ridge Publishing Group
Coeur d'Alene, Idaho, U.S.A.

**DISCLAIMER:** The ideas, concepts, and opinions expressed in The Manhattan Diaries Series (hereinafter referred to as "Series") are intended to help readers make thoughtful and informed decisions about their lifestyle. This Series is sold with the understanding that author and publisher are not rendering medical advice of any kind, nor is this Series intended to replace the medical advice, nor to diagnose, prescribe, or treat any disease, condition, illness, or injury. It should not be used as a substitute for treatment by or the advice of a professional healthcare provider. It is recommended that before beginning any diet or exercise program, including any aspect of the Series, you receive full medical clearance from a licensed healthcare provider. Although the author and publisher have endeavored to ensure that the information provided in the Series is complete and accurate, the author and publisher claim no responsibility to any person or entity for any liability, loss, or damage caused or alleged to be caused directly or indirectly as a result of the use, application, or interpretation of the material in this Series, or any errors or omissions in the Series.

**CREDIT**: This book was written with limited assistance of ChatGPT, an AI language model developed by OpenAI. The collaboration provided unique insights and support in crafting content. The book cover was created using Midjourney tools and Adobe Photoshop, ensuring a visually captivating design.

### Library of Congress Control Number: 2024920974

Urban Elixir: NYC's Proven Blueprint to Timeless Skin / by Jessica Brooks

ISBN: 978-1-956905-23-6 (e-book)
ISBN: 978-1-956905-22-9 (Softcover)

1. Health & Fitness / Beauty & Grooming. 2. Self-Help / Personal Appearance & Grooming. 3. Self-Help / Motivational & Inspirational. 4. Self-Help / Aging. 5. Lifestyle & Personal Style Guides. 6. Self-Help / Happiness.. I. Title. II. Series.

First Edition: September 2024

Printed in the United States of America

# Contents

# The Manhattan Diaries Series

DARE TO REIMAGINE YOURSELF . . .

## 21 Steps to Reinvent and Discover a Side of You Manhattan's Never Seen

The Manhattan Diaries Series presents:

Manhattan Allure—Just Like That mini-series (books 1–5)

Manhattan Vitality—Just Like That mini-series (books 6–10)

Manhattan Lifestyle—Just Like That mini-series (books 11–16)

Manhattan Ambition—Just Like That mini-series (books 17–21)

Meet the Author
https://www.LAMoeszinger.com

Meet the Publisher, Urban Chronicles Publishing House
https://www.NewYouniversityChronicles.com

Step into the whirlwind world of New York's glitzy underbelly, where the scintillating secrets and laugh-out-loud confessions of a metropolitan woman are laid bare by someone truly in the know. Through essays pulled from her chic "Manhattanite's Survival Guide—Success in the City," L invites us on an unforgettable strut from her glamorous youth, through her middle-aged mazes, and into her fabulous sixties.

For the juiciest tidbits about L's life, her "Manhattan Chronicles" blog is the place to be. This blog is an unfiltered dive into L's world, from her spiritual musings to her meticulous weigh-ins to her New Youniversity Chronicles—The Manhattan Diaries series—personal tales. Dive into her cosmos at her blog site: https://www.ManhattanChronicles.com.

The Manhattan Diaries Series

# Urban Elixir
## NYC's Proven Blueprint
## To Timeless Skin

Manhattan Allure
Just Like That

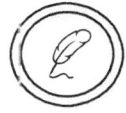

# Introduction: The Manhattan Potion — NYC's Regimen for Eternal Glow

Well, hello there, urban explorers! As you navigate the vibrant streets of New York City, have you ever wondered how its elite maintain their timeless skin amidst the hustle and bustle of the metropolis? Do you stride through the city's concrete canyons with the confidence of a true New Yorker, or are you still deciphering the secrets to achieving ageless skin in the urban jungle? Well, dear readers, the city holds the key to timeless skin, and I'm here to unveil it all in "Urban Elixir: NYC's Proven Blueprint to Timeless Skin."

In this captivating journey, I'm taking you behind the scenes of New York City's skincare connoisseurs. Success in the Big Apple isn't just about wit or navigating its complex streets—it's about possessing skin that defies the passage of time and leaves a lasting impression at every glamorous event, from uptown soirees to downtown gatherings. I've mingled with the city's haut monde, attended exclusive soirees, and unearthed the skincare secrets that keep NYC's finest looking eternally youthful. But remember, true beauty emanates from within.

Consider this your exclusive invitation to a limited-edition of The Manhattan Diaries, experience. Whether you savor this treasure trove over leisurely days, indulge in it week by week, or read it while sipping cocktails on Manhattan rooftops, the pace is entirely up to you. Visualize yourself diving into a chapter with your morning latte or immersing yourself in the entire book during a weekend escape. Within these pages, you'll unlock the keys to becoming the master of your skin care destiny, and the timeless beauty that follows will leave you spellbound.

As we embark on this journey together, I'll be your confidante, revealing how effortlessly you can conquer the world of skin care in the city that never sleeps. This guide isn't just about skin care tips; it's a rejuvenation of your spirit, your relationships, and your aspirations in the city. Join me in uncovering the secrets that will make your skin glow as luminously as the city skyline at twilight. I'm not just dedicated to helping you master the art of timeless skin; I'm here to ignite the confidence in your heart that propels you to your most radiant self. Embrace it, and the energy of New York will be yours to command!

My passion for this city-centric guide is born from my own personal journey, filled with highs and lows, passion and heartbreaks. Like many city dwellers, I had to blaze my own trail, sometimes veering off the well-trodden path. But today, I stand before you, ready to inspire you to conquer your city with your skin as your canvas, cocktail in hand.

As time sails on the Hudson River, our life paths inevitably intersect. For me, the whirlwind of career pursuits, downtown extravaganzas, and self-discovery converged with my love for the city, leading me to work with the Urban Chronicles Publishing House.

New York City's allure isn't limited to celebrities or trust fund beneficiaries; it's accessible to everyone, whether you're a chic twenty-something or a sophisticated sixty-something. Embrace this journey with me as we embark on a path to city stardom in this fifth step—The Manhattan Diaries series is a twenty-one step journey; twenty-one books to reinvent and discover a side of you Manhattan's never met.

"Urban Elixir" equips you with the tools to not only dream big but to seize those dreams. I'm here as your city guardian, ensuring you realize that everything you crave starts within. With this guide, nurture your mind, body, and soul with Manhattan's finest secrets, and watch as your dream job, penthouse, or perfect partner follows suit. If you've got city-sized dreams, this series is your key to unlocking them! I've witnessed friends rise to city stardom time and time again, proving that as you align within, the city will reflect it back in glitz and glamour. That's a promise straight from the heart of New York.

Relying on The Manhattan Diaries series has always been my lifeline. Whenever the city threw a curveball my way, this series steered me right back to my radiant path. The allure of always being at the peak of beauty keeps me coming back to these page, and trust me, it's far more exhilarating than settling for mediocrity.

With every page you turn, you'll discover the blueprint, insider secrets, and the support you need to make your transformative journey an exhilarating adventure. This series is tailored for everyone, from those seeking a fabulous career to social butterflies and empire builders.

There are countless ways to rise in the Big Apple, but if you're looking for the chicest route, it's right here in this city series—The Manhattan Diaries. Immerse yourself in its treasures while reciting positive mantras, and let the city's vibrancy chase away any doubts; and, in this case, allowing yourself to become your unique masterpiece. To truly reign, sometimes we need to shed our old routines and embrace our most radiant selves.

## Navigating the City with The Manhattan Diaries

Welcome to "Urban Elixir: NYC's Proven Blueprint to Timeless Skin." Think of this edition of The Manhattan Diaries as your personal cosmopolitan diary. As interactive as an invitation to Manhattan's most exclusive soirees. Each chapter is enriched with journal pages, waiting for your Manhattan musings and anecdotes. Whether you want to record the day's chic highlights in your "Skin Chronicles" or delve into deep reflections in your "Skin Confessions," these pages are yours to fill—see Cocktails and Chronicles: "Journal Pages: Pen Your Tales."

But . . .

/ Before you start penning your thoughts, take a moment to breathe. Close your eyes and, in that quiet moment, express a heartfelt "thank you" to the city that never sleeps. Feel that rush of gratitude, as if you've just been given a front row seat to New York Fashion Week. Let that "thank you" resonate deep within your heart—because that, my dear readers, is the magic of Manhattan.

2 Begin by detailing the fabulous strides you've made since delving into the last glamorous advice you've received. Write them down under "Completed Tasks," and relish in the feeling of owning every room you walk into with your timeless beauty.

3 Once you've celebrated your skin care triumphs, turn the page, to "Action Items" and outline your aspirations. Reflect on what's left to conquer in your skin care journey, capturing your next steps in this transformational saga.

Throughout The Manhattan Diaries series, you'll encounter timeless "inspirational quotes" that are as iconic as Manhattan's skyline. These pearls of wisdom are your beauty mantras. Savor them, recite each word as if you're toasting at an Upper East Side salon, and let them resonate deep within your urban beauty soul.

As you approach the end of each guide, you'll discover a "City Roundup." Here, you'll find a chic recap summarizing all the insider tips from your beauty escapade, ensuring you never miss a New York beauty minute.

So, get ready to unlock the secrets of Manhattan's timeless beauty elite, darlings. Behind the cityscape lies a world of allure, style, and endless possibilities for your skin. It's time to let your beauty shine as brightly as the city lights.

## Urban Elixir: NYC's Proven Blueprint to Timeless Skin

Prepare to be captivated by the secrets of timeless beauty in the heart of the city with "Urban Elixir: NYC's Proven Blueprint to Timeless Skin," the fifth dazzling chapter in The Manhattan Diaries series. If you're on the quest for a sensational life my dear readers, consider this your next essential step.

In "Urban Elixir," you'll unveil the blueprint to achieving that vibrant, ageless allure that sets you apart in the urban jungle. Imagine skin that defies time, radiating vitality and freshness. They say ninety percent of aging is genetic, but we've got the power to control the other ten percent. Sun avoidance, sunscreen, and bidding farewell to those smoking habits are your allies on this journey.

But here's the secret weapon, darlings; optimism. It's the golden ticket to staying fresh and youthful. In the city that never sleeps, your skin deserves nothing less than a magical elixir of confidence and self-love.

So, join me on this enchanting path where we explore the art of timeless beauty. With "Urban Elixir: NYC's Proven Blueprint to Timeless Skin" as your guide, you'll discover the keys to a vibrant, extraordinary life that leaves you feeling invincible in the city's dazzling lights. Your sensational journey awaits!

## Meet the Maestros Behind the Curtain

Welcome to the glittering realm of The Manhattan Diaries series, penned by an eclectic group of scribes who know how to make words shimmer just like that Midtown skyline. Each of these writers possesses the kind of Manhattan moxie that's as electrifying as a Saturday night at Studio 54. Picture the literary equivalent of the fabulous foursome from "Sex and the City," but with a little extra Manhattan mascara.

Our authors, darlings, aren't just writers; they're connoisseurs of all things NYC, dishing out stories with the precision of a Fifth Avenue stylist crafting the perfect blowout. Their tales are imbued with the kind of insider knowledge only those who've sipped martinis at the city's most secretive spots can truly understand.

So, as you delve into the pages of The Manhattan Diaries know that you're not just reading words, you're sipping on the prose of New York's finest literary mixologists. Here's to a journey as sparkling and unforgettable as a New York night out. Cheers, darling!

## Behind the Scenes with the Urban Chronicles Publishing House

In the whirlwind of New York's high society, the Urban Chronicles Publishing House has emerged as the ultimate style sage for modern-day self-help. Over a cosmopolitan-fueled decade, they've become the city's go-to curators for crafting that sought-after, enviable life. The Manhattan Diaries? Envision it as your exclusive, VIP backstage pass, dripping with Upper East Side allure.

If you've ever pictured yourself sashaying through Manhattan with poise, if you've craved that skyline backdrop to your impeccable life, or if you simply seek the secrets whispered in the plush corners of the city's most exclusive clubs—The Manhattan Diaries is your ticket. Crafted under the elite banner, Urban Chronicles Publishing House, this imprint doesn't just offer you insights; it's your personal invite to the city's most glamorous circles.

> **Forever en Vogue**. Everyone, from the Wall Street moguls to the aspiring Broadway stars, dream of basking in New York's radiant glow, of living a life drenched in style and substance. The wisdom in The Manhattan Diaries is as timeless as a Fifth Avenue romance, ensuring you're always en vogue.

> **A Blueprint for the Elite**. Nestled within these pages are the golden rules of city living, from mastering the cocktail chatter to undergoing a dazzling reinvention. Whether you're a seasoned socialite, an ambitious parent, or a fresh-eyed dreamer, these guides have something to make your heart race a little faster.

> ➤ **The Perfect Accessory.** Their petite stature makes these guides a seamless fit for your Prada clutch or your gym tote. Think of them as your urban survival kit—a blend of wisdom and wit that's as crucial as your red lipstick for those Manhattan nights.

Take a sip of this rich concoction, and let the Urban Chronicles Publishing House unlock Manhattan, unveiling a New York you only dreamed of. Welcome to the allure of the elite, darling.

## Unveiling The Ridge Publishing Group

Picture The Ridge Publishing Group as the rising star on New York's literary and entertainment horizon. Envision an eclectic empire—books, cinema, and board games—setting the stage to become the world's haute couture of theological discourse. Think Fifth Avenue for theological resources: luxurious, elite, and unparalleled.

Dive into their esteemed collections. They hold the keys to the illustrious Guardians of Biblical Truth Publishing Group and the evocative New Narrated Study Bible (NNSB) series. Delve deeper and find the Hoyle Theology Publishing Group and its opulent Hoyle Theology Encyclopedia—a treasure trove for the cerebral sophisticate. And for those who like their theology paired with a cinematic flair, there's the Documentaries in Print Publishing Group with its tantalizing series like Defending the Faith. And, of course, for those cocktail nights with a side of divine strategy, the Heaven's Seminary board games and card decks offer a chic twist.

But that's not all. The Ridge Publishing Group is more than a theological publishing powerhouse; it's a brand. Alongside its flagship, it flaunts trendy imprints: AuthorsDoor Group and the AuthorsDoor Leadership program (check them out at the glamorous digital boulevard of https://www.AuthorsDoor.com), the ritzy Urban Chronicles Publishing House and New Youniversity Chronicles (make your reservation at https://www.NewYouniversityChronicles.com), and the novel delights of

Ethan Fox Books (sip your martini and browse https://www.EthanFox Books.com).

For a sneak peek into the world where theology meets Manhattan glamour, rendezvous at their digital penthouse: https://www.Ridge PublishingGroup.com. It's theology made chic.

## A NOTE TO THE READER

Typos in this book? Errors (and inconsistencies) can get through proofreaders, so if you do find any typos or grammatical errors in this book, I'd be very grateful if you could let me know using this email address typos@LAMoeszinger.com. Thank you ☺

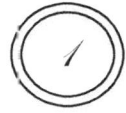

# 1

# Manhattan Mornings: The Wake-Up Rituals for Glowing City Skin

Manhattan, the illustrious city that never truly sleeps. Even in its most muted hours, as the dawn begins to blush over its steel facades, Manhattan stirs, whispers, beckons. It isn't just about enduring the frenzied rhythm of the previous night; it's about awakening with vibrancy, ready to embrace the fresh tales and dreams of a new day—with elegance, zest, and that signature Manhattan panache.

Envision this: As the city stretches and awakens, you're sauntering through Central Park, every ray of morning sun accentuating your radiant complexion. Not one glance is drawn to you because of the designer of your ensemble, but rather the radiant glow of your skin—a luminosity born from the city's morning magic. That, darling, is the Manhattan Morning Marvel, a ritual that whispers tales of rejuvenation, hope, and impeccable grace.

In this refreshing chapter of The Manhattan Diaries, we'll unravel the secrets of that enviable Manhattan morning glow. From the gentle embrace of a hydrating serum to the protective kiss of SPF, you'll learn the intricacies of embracing the city's dawn and ensuring your skin does too, with finesse and luminance.

However, it's more than mere skin care—it's soul care. It's absorbing the essence of Manhattan's dawn, the silent promises whispered by the gentle Hudson waves, and the soft hum of early risers. It's harmonizing with both the serenity of city sunrises and the fervor of what lies ahead, capturing the essence of Manhattan's perpetual hope.

Join me, as we bask in the golden hues of dawn, absorbing the gentle murmurs and vibrant promises, perfecting the art of a morning ritual that illuminates not just your visage, but the very soul of the city. Because in Manhattan, every dawn presents a new narrative, a fresh canvas. Ready yourself, as the city sets the scene for yet another day of dreams and dramas.

Dive deep into The Manhattan Diaries—where your morning radiance rivals the city's first light.

## The Essence of Manhattan's Morning Magic

Picture this, darling: Manhattan at the crack of dawn, a realm where dreams begin to stir, and the city's heartbeat quickens beneath the soft, rosy blush of daybreak. It's a moment dripping with allure, where the enchanting essence of morning magic unfurls like a well-kept secret. This isn't simply about surviving the night's frenetic rhythm; it's about greeting the day with a vibrancy that defines Manhattan-elegance, zest, and that signature panache. Join me on a journey through the captivating essence of Manhattan's morning magic, where every aspect beckons for exploration.

➢ **The City That Never Truly Sleeps**. Manhattan, the vivacious metropolis that laughs in the face of slumber, where its pulse echoes even in the quietest moments. As the dawn breaks, the city's heartbeat persists—a siren's call, an invitation you can't resist. It's an embrace that promises warmth and adventure.

➢ **Awakening to Fresh Tales and Dreams**. Here, each morning unfolds as a pristine canvas, an invitation to script new stories and dreams that await. It's not merely about rousing from slumber; it's about ascending with grace and poise, ready to craft the narrative of the day with your own unique strokes.

➢ **The Radiant Manhattan Morning Glow**. Picture yourself taking a leisurely saunter through Central Park, where the morning sun's tender caress seems to accentuate your luminous complexion. Here, it's not about designer labels; it's about the natural, irresistible glow that comes from being kissed by Manhattan's morning enchantment.

➢ **The Manhattan Morning Marvel**. Now, let's delve into the secrets of attaining that coveted Manhattan morning glow. It's a symphony of skincare artistry, from indulgent hydrating serums to the protective shield of SPF. Each step is a brushstroke on the canvas of your radiant self, transforming your skin into a work of art.

- ➤ **More Than Skin Deep—Soul Care**. But remember, this is more than just skincare; it's soul care-an immersion in the very essence of Manhattan's dawn. It's about harmonizing with the serenity of city sunrises, the gentle hum of early risers, and the enduring hope that defines Manhattan.

- ➤ **Manhattan's Timeless Elegance**. Amidst the morning magic, you'll find Manhattan exuding an unparalleled elegance that transcends time. Its iconic architecture, from Art Deco masterpieces to sleek modern skyscrapers, stands as a testament to the city's enduring allure. It's an atmosphere where sophistication and history intertwine, inviting you to be part of its ongoing narrative.

- ➤ **A Melting Pot of Cultures**. In the early hours, Manhattan is a cultural melting pot, with diverse communities starting their day. From the aromas of freshly brewed coffee in Little Italy to the vibrant colors of street markets in Chinatown, the city's neighborhoods awaken, offering a glimpse into the rich tapestry of cultures that call Manhattan home.

In Manhattan, every dawn is an opportunity to craft fresh narratives, to weave dreams and dramas in a city fueled by ambition and allure. As the city shares its secrets in hushed tones and the sun bathes its iconic skyline, embrace the enchantment of the morning with open arms and an open heart. Here, morning radiance contends with the city's very first light—a journey where style, grace, and boundless spirit take center stage, allowing you to paint the canvas of your day with the vibrant hues of Manhattan's morning magic.

## Completed Tasks: Morning Magic Activities

_____
_____
_____
_____
_____
_____
_____
_____
_____
_____
_____
_____
_____
_____
_____
_____
_____
_____
_____
_____
_____
_____
_____
_____

*Inspirational Quote*

I BELIEVE IN LIVING TODAY. NOT IN YESTERDAY, NOR IN TOMORROW. —
Loretta Young

*Action Items: Intentions and Thoughts*

## *Unlocking the Secrets of Morning Skincare*

Darling, let's dive into a world of morning skincare—a realm where pampering yourself becomes an art, and every ritual is a promise of radiant beauty. It's not just about products and routines; it's about unlocking the secrets to morning skincare, where each step is a brushstroke on the canvas of your own elegance. Join me as we unravel this exquisite tapestry, one skincare secret at a time, in a tone that's as evocative as the city itself.

➢ **The Morning Elixir: The First Sip of Radiance**. Picture this: your first step in the morning, like savoring the first sip of an exquisite elixir. This is where hydration reigns supreme. Hydrating serums infused with potent ingredients become your morning muse, infusing your skin with a luminosity that rivals the city's very skyline.

➢ **The Gentle Awakening: Cleansing as a Morning Ritual**. Cleansing isn't just about removing yesterday's makeup; it's a ritual that awakens your skin. Imagine a gentle cleanse, a moment of purity where your skin breathes. It's the art of starting anew, like the dawn itself.

➢ **Morning Indulgence: The Ritual of Facial Massage**. Visualize the morning as a canvas for self-indulgence. Incorporate a gentle facial massage into your skincare routine. This massage not only enhances blood circulation but also adds a touch of luxury to your morning, leaving your skin looking and feeling rejuvenated.

➢ **Eyes that Speak Volumes: De-puffing and Brightening for a Fresh Gaze**. Your eyes are the windows to your soul, and in Manhattan, they need to shine. Incorporate a de-puffing eye cream and a brightening treatment into your morning routine to ensure your gaze is as fresh and captivating as the city itself.

➢ **The Shield of Protection: Embracing the Power of SPF**. SPF isn't just sunscreen; it's your shield against the city's daily adventures. Envision it as your armor, guarding your radiant canvas from the urban elements. It's about ensuring that your glow remains undiminished throughout the day.

➢ **Hydration from Within: Sip on Morning Elixirs**. The morning is the perfect time to nourish your skin from within. Sip on a morning elixir, such as a cup of antioxidant-rich green tea or a concoction of lemon water with a dash of honey. These elixirs not only hydrate but also detoxify, giving your skin a radiant, healthy glow.

➢ **The Power of a Morning Mindset: Cultivating Positivity**. Don't forget, darling, that skincare goes beyond products—it's a mindset. Start your day with positivity, affirmations, and a smile that radiates confidence. A positive mindset is the ultimate secret to looking and feeling beautiful, no matter what Manhattan has in store for you.

➢ **The Final Flourish: A Touch of Morning Makeup**. Complete your morning skincare symphony with a flourish of makeup. Think of it as the finishing touch on your masterpiece. A subtle stroke of mascara, a hint of blush—each detail enhances your beauty, readying you for whatever the city may bring.

Morning skincare is not just a routine; it's an act of self-care, a daily ritual that mirrors the grace and elegance of the Manhattan mornings. As you unlock the secrets of skincare, envision yourself as an artist, crafting your own canvas of beauty, ready to embrace the world with the confidence and allure of a Manhattanite. It's a journey where every step is a brushstroke, and your radiance rivals the city's first light.

## Completed Tasks: Morning Skincare Activities

_____
_____
_____
_____
_____
_____
_____
_____
_____
_____
_____
_____
_____
_____
_____
_____
_____
_____
_____
_____
_____
_____
_____
_____
_____
_____

*Inspirational Quote*

AND NOW, THIS IS THE SWEETEST AND MOST GLORIOUS DAY THAT EVER MY EYES DID SEE. — Donald Cargill

*Action Items: Intentions and Thoughts*

## Soul Care in the City

Darling, let's delve into the art of soul care in the city—a realm where the heart of Manhattan aligns with your own. In this urban jungle, it's not just about skyscrapers and bustling streets; it's about nurturing your inner self amidst the chaos and allure. Join me as we explore the delicate dance of soul care in the city, where every step is a journey into the very essence of Manhattan's perpetual hope, in a voice as evocative as the city lights.

➤ **Harmonizing with City Sunrises**. Visualize the dawn breaking over the city's skyline—an exquisite moment of serenity amid the urban hustle. Wake early, bask in the gentle embrace of the morning sun, and let the tranquility of city sunrises wash over you. It's about finding peace in the midst of city chaos.

➤ **Whispers of the Hudson: Communing with Nature in the Urban Jungle**. Imagine a stroll along the Hudson River, where the soft whispers of the waves become a soothing symphony. Amidst the city's concrete jungle, find solace in nature's embrace, letting the river's rhythm connect you to the city's enduring spirit.

➤ **The Morning Playlist: Music for the Soul**. Envision a playlist curated to accompany your morning rituals—a selection of songs that resonate with your spirit. Allow music to infuse your soul with inspiration, elevating your morning routine to a harmonious crescendo that mirrors Manhattan's vibrant energy.

➤ **City Streets as Meditation Paths: Finding Tranquility Amidst the Chaos**. Consider the city streets as your meditation paths, where the bustling chaos becomes a backdrop for inner serenity. Take a leisurely walk, focus on your breath, and let the urban rhythms guide you towards a sense of calm, even in the heart of Manhattan's vibrant streets.

- ➤ **Artistic Escapades: Immerse in Urban Art and Culture** Indulge your soul in Manhattan's rich art and cultural scene. Visit galleries, theaters, or simply admire the street art adorning the city's walls. Immerse yourself in the creative spirit of Manhattan, where every piece of art tells a story and feeds your inner muse.

- ➤ **Culinary Adventures: Savor the City's Flavors**. Soul care extends to your taste buds. Explore Manhattan's diverse culinary offerings, from street vendors to Michelin-starred restaurants. Savor the flavors of the city, indulging in delectable meals that nourish not just your body but your spirit as well.

- ➤ **Connecting with Kindred Spirits: Building Community in the Urban Maze**. In the city that never sleeps, building connections with kindred spirits is essential for soul care. Attend meetups, join clubs, or engage in communal activities that resonate with your interests. In this vast metropolis, you'll find your tribe, a supportive community that nurtures your soul amidst the city's dynamism.

- ➤ **The City's Perpetual Hope: Embracing Optimism**. Lastly, remember that soul care in the city is also about nurturing your spirit with the city's perpetual hope. Manhattan thrives on ambition and dreams. Embrace its optimism, let it fuel your aspirations, and allow it to be the beacon guiding your soul through the urban labyrinth.

In the heart of Manhattan, amidst the skyscrapers and bustling streets, lies a realm where soul care becomes an art—a delicate dance between embracing the city's chaos and finding solace in its beauty. As you harmonize with city sunrises, commune with nature, and let music serenade your soul, you'll discover that Manhattan's essence is not just perpetual hope; it's an invitation to nurture your inner self in the most evocative way. It's a journey where the rhythm of your soul resonates with the vibrant heartbeat of the city, creating a harmony that's uniquely Manhattan.

## Completed Tasks: Soul Care Activities

_____
_____
_____
_____
_____
_____
_____
_____
_____
_____
_____
_____
_____
_____
_____
_____
_____
_____
_____
_____
_____
_____
_____
_____
_____
_____
_____
_____
_____
_____
_____
_____

### Inspirational Quote

FROM WHAT WE GET, WE CAN MAKE A LIVING; WHAT WE GIVE, HOWEVER,
MAKES A LIFE. — Arthur Ashe

*Action Items: Intentions and Thoughts*

## Embracing Manhattan's Perpetual Hope

Darling, let's dive into the boundless optimism that is Manhattan's perpetual hope—a city where dreams are woven into the very fabric of existence. In this bustling metropolis, hope is not just an emotion; it's a way of life, a driving force that propels you forward amidst the ceaseless energy of the city. Join me as we embrace the essence of Manhattan's perpetual hope, in a voice as evocative as the city's skyline at sunset.

> ➤ **The City That Inspires Dreams**. Manhattan, the city that inspires dreams like no other. It's a place where every corner holds the promise of a new beginning, where ambition fuels aspirations, and where the skyline is a testament to the heights one can reach. In Manhattan, hope is as ubiquitous as the skyscrapers that define its silhouette.

> ➤ **The Art of Reinvention: Writing Your Own Story**. Visualize Manhattan as a canvas, a place where you can reinvent yourself. Here, hope is the brush, and you are the artist. Embrace the art of reinvention, where the city encourages you to write your own story, unburdened by the past and limitless in possibility.

> ➤ **The Thrill of Possibility: Navigating Uncertainty with Grace**. In the city that never sleeps, uncertainty is a constant companion. But rather than fear it, envision uncertainty as a thrilling ride, an adventure waiting to be embraced. Manhattan's perpetual hope lies in your ability to navigate uncertainty with grace, knowing that each twist and turn can lead to new opportunities.

> ➤ **The Magnetic Pull of Ambition: Fueling Your Drive**. Manhattan's perpetual hope is also found in its magnetic pull of ambition. In this city, ambition is not seen as a flaw but as a beacon, a guiding light that propels you forward. It's the recognition that

your dreams are not just valid but attainable, no matter how audacious they may be.

➢ **The Resilient Spirit of Manhattanites: Inspiring Stories of Triumph**. Consider the resilient spirit of Manhattanites, the individuals who have weathered storms and emerged stronger than ever. Their stories of triumph in the face of adversity become a wellspring of hope, reminding you that resilience is a badge of honor in this city.

➢ **Cultural Kaleidoscope: Embracing Diversity as a Source of Strength**. In Manhattan, diversity isn't just tolerated; it's celebrated. The multitude of cultures, backgrounds, and perspectives is a testament to the city's open-mindedness. Embrace this cultural kaleidoscope as a source of strength, recognizing that unity through diversity is a powerful manifestation of hope.

➢ **The Magic of Serendipity: Embracing Unexpected Opportunities**. Lastly, Manhattan's perpetual hope resides in the magic of serendipity. It's the belief that around every corner, unexpected opportunities await. In this city of chance encounters and serendipitous moments, hope thrives, reminding you to always be open to the possibility of the extraordinary.

As you walk the streets of Manhattan, let the city's perpetual hope seep into your soul. It's an invitation to dream, to reinvent, to embrace uncertainty, and to fuel your drive with unapologetic ambition. In the heart of this metropolis, hope is not just a sentiment; it's the very air you breathe, the pulse that keeps the city alive. It's a reminder that in Manhattan, the possibilities are as limitless as the sky, and your dreams are always within reach, waiting to be realized in the most evocative way possible.

## Completed Tasks: Perpetual Hope Activities

_____
_____
_____
_____
_____
_____
_____
_____
_____
_____
_____
_____
_____
_____
_____
_____
_____
_____
_____
_____
_____
_____
_____
_____
_____
_____

### Inspirational Quote

KEEP ALL SPECIAL THOUGHTS AND MEMORIES FOR LIFETIMES TO COME. SHARE THESE KEEPSAKES WITH OTHERS TO INSPIRE HOPE AND BUILD FROM THE PAST, WHICH CAN BRIDGE TO THE FUTURE. — Mattie Stepanek

# MANHATTAN MORNINGS

*Action Items: Intentions and Thoughts*

*Action Items: Intentions and Thoughts*

# 2

# SoHo Serums: The Magic Potions Every New Yorker Swears By

Manhattan, a city drenched in a cocktail of dreams, aspirations, and those insatiable desires to be seen, felt, and remembered. Each cobblestone and skyscraper vibrates with tales of moxie, ambition, and the undeniable allure of transformation. Navigating this urban wonder isn't just about plotting a path—it's about charting a journey rife with flair, finesse, and that undeniable Manhattan mystique.

Picture this: You're cruising through the artistic heart of SoHo, every gaze inexplicably captivated, not by the designer tag of your ensemble, but by the mesmerizing luminance of your skin. That glow, my darling, is the magic of SoHo Serums, the city's best-kept secret—a testament to resilience, renewal, and that exquisite Manhattan reinvention.

In this alluring chapter of The Manhattan Diaries, we delve into the mystique behind these coveted elixirs. From the transformative droplets that promise age-defiance to the invigorating potions that breathe life into tired complexions, you'll uncover the allure of these bottled wonders, a love affair known only to those truly in tune with the city's pulse.

Yet, it's not just about topical transformation. It's a romance with the city's essence, a dance with its ever-evolving rhythm. It's about infusing one's very being with the spirit of SoHo's art, passion, and the timeless tales whispered between its historic walls. It's mastering the delicate balance between the artistry of self-presentation and the raw, unabashed self beneath.

So, join me, as we explore the alchemy of these SoHo enchantments, imbibing the secrets that have, for ages, maintained Manhattan's ageless allure. Because in this city of dreams, reinvention isn't just a choice—it's a lifestyle. Ready yourself, for the city beckons with a new tale, a new promise. Step into The Manhattan Diaries—where your glow is as enigmatic as the city's most intimate secrets.

## The Allure of SoHo Serums

Darling, let's delve into the irresistible allure of SoHo Serums—the unspoken obsession of every savvy New Yorker. In the heart of Manhattan, where desires and aspirations intersect, these serums weave a tale of ageless allure and the promise of transformative beauty. Picture the cobblestone streets and loft apartments of SoHo, where artistry meets sophistication, and these serums take center stage. Join me in uncovering the secrets behind the captivating essence of SoHo Serums, in a voice as evocative as the city lights at twilight.

> ➢ **The Manhattan Enigma**. In this ever-pulsating city, where dreams materialize in the blink of an eye, SoHo Serums reflect the essence of Manhattan—a place where aspirations and ambition intertwine, creating a tapestry of desires and timeless allure.

> ➢ **The Elixir of Radiance**. Enter the world of SoHo Serums, where science meets artistry to promise age-defying, luminous skin. These elixirs are more than mere beauty products; they hold the power to captivate, leaving an indelible mark on those who dare to indulge.

> ➢ **SoHo's Influence on Self-Presentation**. SoHo isn't just a neighborhood; it's a mindset—a place where personal style and self-expression reign supreme. In the artistic and sophisticated atmosphere of SoHo, the allure of these serums enhances one's self-presentation, creating a magnetic aura that draws admirers.

> ➢ **The Balance of Artistry and Authenticity**. In the city that never sleeps, the art of self-presentation is a delicate dance. SoHo Serums play a pivotal role in this performance, not as masks but as enhancers of inner confidence. They are the bridge between artistry and authenticity, helping individuals find the perfect balance.

➤ **The Ritual of Self-Care**. SoHo Serums represent a daily ritual of self-care—a moment to pamper oneself amidst the city's bustling energy, a reminder that you are worthy of the utmost attention and care.

➤ **A Glowing Emblem of Confidence**. Using these serums isn't just about enhancing your appearance; it's about radiating confidence. Picture the self-assured stride of a New Yorker, knowing that their luminance is more than skin-deep.

➤ **SoHo as a Lifestyle Influence**. SoHo Serums are a testament to SoHo's influence on lifestyle and fashion. They encapsulate the neighborhood's artistic flair, setting a trend of sophistication and self-expression.

➤ **The Intrigue of Discreet Luxury**. Much like Manhattan itself, these serums exude a sense of discreet luxury—a whispered secret among those in the know. They offer an exclusive experience, adding to the city's mystique and allure.

➤ **The Legacy of Timeless Elegance.** SoHo Serums not only offer a contemporary touch to beauty regimes but also draw on the rich heritage of SoHo's historical elegance. Each drop carries the legacy of decades, blending modern scientific breakthroughs with the timeless charm that the SoHo district is renowned for.

As you navigate the streets of SoHo, let the allure of SoHo Serums seep into your very soul. They embody more than just beauty; they encapsulate the spirit of Manhattan—a relentless pursuit of excellence, an eternal quest for allure, and a celebration of ageless beauty. Amidst the cobblestone and couture, embrace the essence of these serums, for within their transformative power lies the key to unlocking your own Manhattan mystique.

*Completed Tasks: SoHo Serums Activities*

_____

_____

_____

_____

_____

_____

_____

_____

_____

_____

_____

_____

_____

_____

_____

_____

_____

_____

_____

_____

_____

_____

_____

_____

_____

_____

*Inspirational Quote*

LIVE YOUR BELIEFS AND YOU CAN TURN THE WORLD AROUND. — Henry David Thoreau

# SOHO SERUMS

*Action Items: Intentions and Thoughts*

## The Art of Reinvention in Manhattan

Darling, let's take a stroll through the ever-evolving streets of Manhattan—a city where reinvention isn't just an idea; it's a way of life. Amidst the towering skyscrapers and bustling avenues, Manhattanites have perfected the art of reinvention—a captivating dance between self-expression and transformation. Imagine a skyline that mirrors the aspirations of countless souls, where ambition reigns supreme, and change is the only constant. Join me as we explore the essence of reinvention in Manhattan, in a voice as evocative as the city's twinkling lights at twilight.

- **The Manhattan Metamorphosis**. In this concrete jungle, every day is an opportunity for a Manhattan metamorphosis. The city's dynamic environment fuels personal growth and reinvention, pushing individuals to embrace change with open arms.

- **Reinvention Through Style**. Personal style becomes a potent tool in the art of reinvention, where fashion serves as a canvas for self-expression. Manhattanites use clothing and accessories to craft their evolving identities, reflecting their inner transformations in the way they present themselves to the world.

- **Cultural Evolution in the City**. Manhattan's vibrant cultural scene encourages reinvention through diverse experiences. From exploring new hobbies to immersing in different neighborhoods and communities, the city's cultural melting pot offers endless opportunities for personal growth and change.

- **The Power of Reinvention as a Lifestyle**. Reinvention isn't a sporadic choice in Manhattan; it's a lifestyle embraced by its residents. The pursuit of self-improvement and growth is a constant, fueled by the unshakable belief in the city's boundless possibilities.

- ➤ **The Reinvention of Ambition**. In Manhattan, reinvention isn't limited to personal style or hobbies; it extends to careers and ambitions. The city's competitive spirit drives individuals to constantly reinvent their professional paths, seeking new heights and conquering uncharted territories.

- ➤ **The Role of Resilience**. Reinvention often requires resilience, and in Manhattan, resilience is a prized attribute. It's the ability to bounce back from setbacks, adapt to change, and emerge stronger—a key to success in a city that never stops moving.

- ➤ **The Magnetic Pull of Manhattan**. Explore the magnetic pull of Manhattan, where the allure of reinvention draws dreamers and visionaries from around the world. This irresistible force makes the city a perpetual hub for those seeking personal and professional transformation.

- ➤ **Reinvention as an Ongoing Narrative**. In the narrative of Manhattan, reinvention is not a singular event but an ongoing saga. It's a tale of constant evolution, a journey where the next chapter promises new beginnings and unforeseen adventures, making the city's story as captivating as the lives of its inhabitants.

As you navigate the labyrinthine streets of Manhattan, absorb the art of reinvention that permeates the very air. Here, change isn't feared; it's welcomed as a chance to redefine oneself. The city's ever-evolving nature is a wellspring of inspiration, a daily reminder that you possess the power to recreate yourself. In this dynamic metropolis, reinvention isn't merely an option; it's the heartbeat of the city, an ongoing masterpiece where the canvas is as limitless as the skyline itself. Step into The Manhattan Diaries, where transformation is an art, and the possibilities are boundless.

## Completed Tasks: Reinvention Activities

_____
_____
_____
_____
_____
_____
_____
_____
_____
_____
_____
_____
_____
_____
_____
_____
_____
_____
_____
_____
_____
_____
_____
_____
_____
_____
_____
_____

_Inspirational Quote_

EVERYONE HERE HAS THE SENSE THAT RIGHT NOW IS ONE OF THOSE
MOMENTS WHEN WE ARE INFLUENCING THE FUTURE. — Steve Jobs

*Action Items: Intentions and Thoughts*

*Unveiling the Secrets of SoHo Elixirs*

Darling, let's embark on a covert journey into the depths of SoHo, where the streets whisper secrets and loft apartments hold enigmatic allure. In this captivating chapter, we'll unveil the secrets of SoHo Elixirs—a treasure trove promising age-defiance and rejuvenation. Picture the vibrant streets resonating with artistic inspiration; in the midst of it all, these elixirs are the keys to timeless allure. Join me as we unravel the enigmatic world of SoHo Elixirs, in a voice as seductive as a SoHo night ablaze with creativity.

➢ **The Elixir of Youthful Luminance**. Explore the captivating allure of SoHo Elixirs, promising to defy time and bestow luminosity. Delve into the science and artistry behind these elixirs, revealing the secrets of their transformative prowess.

➢ **The Art of Rejuvenation**. Uncover the elixirs' ability to breathe life into tired complexions, reviving and invigorating the skin. Consider the age-old rituals and innovative science that converge to create these revitalizing concoctions.

➢ **SoHo's Alchemical Influence**. Explore how SoHo's spirit infuses itself into these elixirs, transforming them into more than beauty products but works of art. Consider the symbiotic relationship between the elixirs and the neighborhood's creative essence, resulting in an alchemical blend of beauty and artistry.

➢ **The Seductive Dance of Transformation**. Delve into the essence of transformation inspired by SoHo Elixirs, where every application becomes a sensuous dance. Highlight how these elixirs aren't just about external beauty but also inner transformation, infusing confidence and allure.

➢ **The SoHo Lifestyle Enhancement**. Consider how SoHo Elixirs seamlessly integrate into the SoHo lifestyle, becoming more than skincare but a symbol of the neighborhood's vibrant culture. Highlight how these elixirs elevate one's daily routine, adding a touch of sophistication and artistry to the mundane.

➢ **Sculpting Beauty, Elevating Confidence**. Explore how SoHo Elixirs empower individuals not just to enhance their appearance but also to boost their confidence. Consider the transformative effect these elixirs have on self-esteem, creating a sense of empowerment and allure.

➢ **SoHo's Enigmatic Allure Unveiled**. Delve into how SoHo Elixirs offer a glimpse into the enigmatic allure of the neighborhood itself, capturing its essence in each drop. Highlight the resonance between these elixirs and the captivating aura of SoHo, making them a cherished secret of those in the know.

➢ **The Elixir of Timeless Beauty**. Explore the idea that these elixirs are more than just temporary fixes; they represent a pursuit of ageless beauty. Consider how they become a part of a broader narrative of maintaining allure and grace over time, mirroring the enduring spirit of SoHo itself.

As you wander the labyrinthine streets of SoHo, allow the secrets of these elixirs to seep into your very being. They are more than mere potions; they embody SoHo's spirit—a fusion of artistic fervor, innovation, and the quest for timeless beauty. Amidst this neighborhood, where creativity flows like a river, embrace the essence of these elixirs. For within their transformative touch lies the key to unlocking your inner and outer allure. In the world of SoHo Elixirs, beauty's mysteries are unveiled, and the secrets of eternal allure are whispered, poised to adorn your life like an ongoing masterpiece.

## Completed Tasks: Elixir Secrets Activities

_Inspirational Quote_

ENTHUSIASM MOVES THE WORLD. —— Arthur Balfour

SOHO SERUMS

*Action Items: Intentions and Thoughts*

## *SoHo's Influence on Personal Expression*

Darling, let's dive into the captivating world of SoHo, where the streets themselves seem to whisper fashion secrets and every boutique window is a stage for self-expression. In this enchanting chapter, we'll explore how SoHo's unique ambiance shapes individual style and personal expression. Picture the cobblestone streets as a bustling runway, and each passerby a character in their own fashion narrative. Join me in unraveling the magnetic allure of SoHo and its profound impact on personal expression, all in a voice as seductive as the city's twinkling lights at dusk.

➢ **SoHo's Fashion Playground**. SoHo serves as a playground for fashion aficionados, where sartorial experimentation knows no bounds. The neighborhood's eclectic boutiques and avant-garde galleries play a pivotal role in shaping distinctive personal styles.

➢ **The Bohemian Spirit**. SoHo's bohemian spirit fosters an atmosphere of freedom and encourages unconventional fashion choices. Boho-chic reigns supreme, intertwined with the neighborhood's artistic essence, inspiring a relaxed yet sophisticated flair.

➢ **A Canvas for Self-Expression**. SoHo streets become a vibrant canvas for self-expression, where fashion becomes a medium for communication. Clothing, accessories, and even street art are vehicles through which individuals convey their unique personalities and aspirations.

➢ **SoHo's Timeless Inspirations**. Explore how SoHo's unique blend of history and modernity provides a timeless wellspring of inspiration for personal expression. Discuss how elements of the neighborhood's rich past can be seamlessly integrated into contemporary styles, creating a sense of cultural continuity.

➢ **Influence Beyond Fashion**. SoHo's influence transcends mere fashion; it permeates lifestyle, attitudes, and creative pursuits. The neighborhood's vibrant culture inspires residents and visitors alike to express themselves in diverse aspects of life.

➢ **Icons of Individuality**. Highlight the trendsetters and style icons who have emerged from SoHo, shaping fashion movements and setting the stage for self-expression. Consider how these luminaries continue to influence personal style, making SoHo a breeding ground for trendsetters.

➢ **Cultural Fusion and Self-Discovery**. Delve into how the cultural diversity of SoHo encourages self-discovery and the fusion of different fashion elements. Explore how individuals draw from various cultural influences to craft unique and hybrid styles reflective of their own journeys.

➢ **Art as a Catalyst for Expression**. Examine the profound connection between art and personal expression in SoHo, where galleries, street art, and installations inspire both fashion choices and creative self-discovery. Consider how artistic expressions become an integral part of personal style, making SoHo a true haven for artistic souls.

As you traverse the enchanting streets of SoHo, allow its influence on personal expression to seep into your very soul. Here, individuality is celebrated, and self-expression is an art form. Amidst this neighborhood where creativity knows no boundaries, embrace the essence of SoHo's fashion playground and let it ignite your unique style. Whether you're embracing the latest runway trends or curating vintage treasures, remember that SoHo's allure is an ever-present muse. Step into the world of SoHo, where personal expression becomes a living masterpiece, and every day is an opportunity to craft your own vibrant narrative.

## Completed Tasks: Personal Expression Activities

_____
_____
_____
_____
_____
_____
_____
_____
_____
_____
_____
_____
_____
_____
_____
_____
_____
_____
_____
_____
_____
_____
_____
_____
_____
_____
_____
_____

_Inspirational Quote_

WHAT WE THINK, WE BECOME. — Buddha

# Action Items: Intentions and Thoughts

## Action Items: Intentions and Thoughts

# 3

# Met Gala Masks: Indulgent Treatments for an Event-Ready Complexion

Manhattan, the epicenter of dreams, drama, and decadence, where every pavement reverberates with stories of glory, grit, and unabashed glamour. Here, it's not just about tracing the city's grid; it's about owning every inch of it—with elegance, eloquence, and that signature Manhattan éclat.

Envision this: You're making your entrance at the steps of the Met, not merely as an attendee but as the night's radiant muse. It's not your couture gown that's the talk of the town, but the porcelain perfection of your complexion. That, darling, is the Met Gala Glow, an emblem of finesse, luxury, and a dalliance with the city's crème de la crème skin care rituals.

In this tantalizing installment of The Manhattan Diaries, we'll pull back the velvet curtain on the secrets to achieving that gala-ready radiance. From the opulent masks infused with gold leaf to the transformative treatments favored by the Manhattan elite, you're about to embark on an indulgent journey to luminous, red carpet worthy skin.

But this saga isn't merely skin-deep. It's a dance with the city's ethos—a blend of timeless elegance and forward-thinking innovation. It's about recognizing the masterpiece within, letting it shimmer beneath the city lights, and basking in both the grandeur of the Met and the allure of the moonlit Manhattan skyline.

So, come along, as we immerse ourselves in the rituals that have graced the faces of the city's royalty. Because, sweetheart, in the world of Manhattan glamour, every evening holds the promise of an epic tale, and every face tells a story. Ready to dazzle? The city's grandest soiree awaits your grand reveal. Dive into The Manhattan Diaries—where your glow rivals the city's most illustrious stars.

## The Met Gala Glow: Unveiling the Epitome of Radiance

Darling, let's step into the dazzling world of Manhattan, where every night holds the promise of an epic tale and beauty becomes an exquisite art. In this captivating chapter of The Manhattan Diaries, we unveil the secrets of the Met Gala Glow—a beacon of finesse, luxury, and the city's crème de la crème skincare rituals. Picture yourself ascending the steps of the Met, not just as an attendee, but as the night's radiant muse. It's not your couture gown that's the talk of the town, but the porcelain perfection of your complexion. Join me as we pull back the velvet curtain and embark on an indulgent journey to luminous, red carpet-worthy skin, all in a voice as enchanting as the city lights at dusk.

> ➢ **The Allure of the Met Gala Glow**. In the enchanting world of Manhattan, the Met Gala Glow reigns supreme, where a flawless complexion takes precedence over couture gowns. Attendees at this illustrious event become radiant muses, their skin an epitome of finesse and luxury. As the city's beauty secrets unfold, one realizes that the Met Gala isn't just a soiree; it's an ode to luminous, red carpet-worthy skin.

> ➢ **Opulent Masks: Gilding the Path to Radiance**. Here in Manhattan, skincare is elevated to an art form with opulent masks infused with gold leaf and other decadent ingredients, a favored indulgence of the city's elite. These masks transform beauty routines into luxurious rituals, offering a taste of extravagance and self-pampering that is quintessentially Manhattan.

> ➢ **Red Carpet-Ready Transformations**. Behind the scenes, Manhattan's finest prepare for red carpet events like the Met Gala with transformative skincare treatments that leave skin luminous and event-ready. Cutting-edge innovations and techniques are employed to ensure that each face shines as brilliantly as the city lights.

➢ **Manhattan's Ethos of Elegance and Innovation**. Beyond the surface, these skincare rituals mirror Manhattan's ethos—a fusion of timeless elegance and forward-thinking innovation. It's about recognizing the masterpiece within, letting it shimmer beneath the city lights, and basking in both the grandeur of the Met and the allure of the moonlit Manhattan skyline. In The Manhattan Diaries, your glow rivals the city's most illustrious stars, and every face tells a story in this world where beauty is an art and each evening holds the promise of an epic tale.

➢ **Captivating Met Gala Moments**. At the Met Gala, it's not just about radiant skin but also the moments of sheer magic it creates. Explore the captivating instances where the Met Gala Glow has left a lasting impression, turning attendees into legends of Manhattan's beauty lore.

➢ **The Rituals of Manhattan's Elite**. Dive deeper into the private skincare rituals of Manhattan's elite, discovering the carefully guarded treatments and products that keep their complexions flawless. Uncover the nuances of their regimens and the lengths they go to in pursuit of Met Gala perfection.

As you traverse the enchanting streets of SoHo, allow its influence on personal expression to seep into your very soul. Here, individuality is celebrated, and self-expression is an art form. Amidst this neighborhood where creativity knows no boundaries, embrace the essence of SoHo's fashion playground and let it ignite your unique style. Whether you're embracing the latest runway trends or curating vintage treasures, remember that SoHo's allure is an ever-present muse. Step into the world of SoHo, where personal expression becomes a living masterpiece, and every day is an opportunity to craft your own vibrant narrative.

*Completed Tasks: Met Gala Glow Activities*

_____
_____
_____
_____
_____
_____
_____
_____
_____
_____
_____
_____
_____
_____
_____
_____
_____
_____
_____
_____
_____
_____
_____
_____
_____

*Inspirational Quote*

IT IS NOT IGNORANCE BUT KNOWLEDGE WHICH IS THE MOTHER OF WONDER. — Joseph Wood Krutch

*Action Items: Intentions and Thoughts*

## *Masked in Luxury: Opulent Skincare Rituals*

Darling, let's delve into the opulent world of Manhattan, where beauty becomes an art form and skincare rituals are nothing short of extravagant. In this enchanting chapter, we'll uncover the secrets of opulent skincare rituals that are favored by the city's elite. Picture yourself indulging in masks infused with gold leaf and decadent ingredients, a taste of extravagance that is quintessentially Manhattan. Join me on this journey as we explore the luxurious side of skincare, all in a voice as seductive as the city's twinkling lights at dusk.

➤ **Gilded Elixirs of Beauty**. Here in Manhattan, skincare is transformed into a lavish affair with opulent masks. These masks, often infused with precious gold leaf, pearls, and exotic botanicals, are the crown jewels of beauty regimens. Consider how these masks elevate self-pampering to an art form, embodying the city's penchant for luxury and indulgence.

➤ **The Ritual of Radiance**. Uncover the allure of the skincare ritual itself—a decadent dance of cleansing, exfoliating, and masking, designed to reveal a luminous complexion. Explore the meticulous steps involved in this opulent process, where each movement is an ode to self-care and refinement.

➤ **The Price of Opulence**. Delve into the exclusivity and indulgence associated with opulent skincare. These masks and rituals often come with a hefty price tag, reflecting the city's commitment to extravagance. Consider the allure of investing in oneself, even at a premium, and how it aligns with Manhattan's ethos of self-worth and indulgence.

➤ **Celebrity Inspirations: Icons of Elegance**. Dive into the stories of Manhattan's beauty icons who swear by these luxurious skincare rituals. Explore how celebrities and socialites integrate these extravagant treatments into their routines, setting trends and elevating the standards of skincare luxury.

➢ **Seasonal Sensations: Tailored for Every Climate**. Examine how these opulent skincare rituals adapt to the changing seasons in Manhattan. From summer-specific hydration masks to winter protection elixirs, each treatment is meticulously designed to suit the environmental needs, ensuring year-round radiance and protection.

➢ **Sustainability Meets Luxury**. Discuss the emerging trend of sustainable luxury in skincare. Despite their lavish nature, many high-end Manhattan spas and brands are embracing eco-friendly practices, sourcing ethically obtained ingredients, and featuring biodegradable packaging, merging opulence with environmental consciousness.

➢ **Global Influence: Manhattan's Worldwide Beauty Footprint**. Look at how Manhattan's luxurious skincare trends influence and set standards globally. Think how these opulent rituals have inspired international beauty markets, from Paris to Tokyo, spreading Manhattan's ethos of indulgent beauty across continents.

➢ **Boutique Spa Collaborations: Tailored Luxury Skincare**. Discover the unique collaborations between high-end skincare brands and Manhattan's boutique spas, offering customized treatment experiences that blend expert care with innovative products for a truly luxurious skincare regime.

As you immerse yourself in the world of opulent skincare rituals, remember that here in Manhattan, beauty is not just skin deep; it's an extravagant affair. These masks, infused with opulence, are not mere products—they are symbols of the city's unapologetic love for luxury. Step into The Manhattan Diaries, where beauty becomes a sumptuous dance of refinement and radiance, and where indulgence is a celebration of self-worth.

## Completed Tasks: Skincare Ritual Activities

_____
_____
_____
_____
_____
_____
_____
_____
_____
_____
_____
_____
_____
_____
_____
_____
_____
_____
_____
_____
_____
_____
_____

### Inspirational Quote

WHEN WE SEEK TO DISCOVER THE BEST IN OTHERS, WE SOMEHOW BRING OUT THE BEST IN OURSELVES. — William Arthur Ward

*Action Items: Intentions and Thoughts*

## *Behind the Velvet Curtain: Red Carpet-Ready Transformations*

Darling, let's venture into the glamorous heart of Manhattan, where beauty becomes an exquisite art, and the pursuit of perfection knows no bounds. In this tantalizing chapter, we lift the velvet curtain to reveal the secrets of red carpet-ready transformations—rituals that prepare Manhattan's finest for the most illustrious events, like the Met Gala. Picture yourself behind the scenes, where every face is sculpted to luminous perfection, and every step is a dance of elegance. Join me on this journey as we explore the meticulous techniques and innovations that ensure skin is ready to dazzle under the city's sparkling lights.

> - **The Art of Pre-Event Skincare**. Delve into the art of pre-event skincare, a process where every step is carefully choreographed to reveal flawless, event-ready skin. Explore the importance of cleansing, exfoliating, and nourishing the skin in the days leading up to the grand soiree, reflecting the city's obsession with excellence.

> - **Airbrushed Beauty: Makeup Techniques for the Red Carpet**. Uncover the makeup techniques employed by Manhattan's makeup artists, transforming faces into works of art. Consider the secrets behind airbrushed beauty and how makeup becomes a tool of self-expression and confidence on the red carpet.

> - **Innovations in Event-Ready Skincare**. Highlight the cutting-edge innovations and treatments that Manhattan's elite indulge in to ensure their skin is at its prime for high-profile events. From non-invasive procedures to the latest in skincare technology, explore the lengths to which these individuals go to achieve red carpet perfection.

> - **The Transformation Experience: Beyond the Surface**. Beyond skincare and makeup, discuss the transformative experience itself. Attending a high-profile event in Manhattan is not just about

appearances; it's about embodying confidence, elegance, and the city's ethos of grandeur. Explore how red carpet transformations extend beyond the surface, becoming a celebration of self-assurance and the allure of Manhattan's glamorous world.

➢ **Luxury Skin Treatments and Spas**. Discover the exclusive spas and luxury treatments that play a crucial role in preparing Manhattan's elite for the red carpet. Delve into the opulent offerings like gold facials, caviar creams, and diamond peels that not only promise radiant skin but also an indulgent experience that starts the glamour long before the event.

➢ **Personal Style Coaches and Image Consultants**. Explore the behind-the-scenes influence of personal style coaches and image consultants who curate each aspect of an attendee's red carpet appearance. These professionals ensure that every detail, from attire to accessories, complements the individual's persona and enhances their overall presence at high-profile gatherings.

➢ **Psychological Preparation for the Spotlight**. Analyze the often-overlooked aspect of mental and emotional preparation that goes into red carpet appearances. Learn about the techniques that help stars maintain composure and exude confidence in the face of overwhelming media attention and public scrutiny.

As you immerse yourself in the world of red carpet-ready transformations, remember that here in Manhattan, perfection is not just an ideal; it's an art form. These rituals, meticulously designed to bring out the best in every individual, reflect the city's passion for excellence and the belief that every step towards beauty is a step towards self-assurance. Step into The Manhattan Diaries, where red carpet readiness becomes a journey of elegance and confidence, and where every face shines as brilliantly as the city's stars.

## Completed Tasks: Transformation Activities

_____
_____
_____
_____
_____
_____
_____
_____
_____
_____
_____
_____
_____
_____
_____
_____
_____
_____
_____
_____
_____
_____
_____
_____
_____
_____
_____
_____
_____
_____

### Inspirational Quote

IF YOU COULD ONLY LOVE ENOUGH, YOU COULD BE THE MOST POWERFUL PERSON IN THE WORLD. — Emmet Fox

*Action Items: Intentions and Thoughts*

## *Manhattan's Ethos of Elegance and Innovation*

Darling, let's journey deep into the heart of Manhattan, where beauty isn't just a facade, but an art form that radiates from within. In this captivating chapter, we'll explore Manhattan's ethos of elegance and innovation, where the pursuit of excellence extends far beyond the surface. Picture a city that thrives on pushing boundaries, embracing new ideas, and celebrating the extraordinary. Join me on this enlightening voyage as we uncover how Manhattan's elite embody both timeless elegance and forward-thinking innovation, all in a voice as enchanting as the city lights at twilight.

➤ **Elegance: A Timeless Manhattan Virtue**. Delve into the timeless virtue of elegance that defines Manhattan's social elite. Explore how elegance isn't just about appearances; it's a way of life that encompasses grace, refinement, and an unwavering commitment to sophistication.

➤ **Innovation: The City's Ever-Evolving Beat**. Unveil Manhattan's insatiable appetite for innovation, a trait that propels the city forward. Consider how innovation touches every aspect of Manhattan life, from fashion and technology to culture and beauty.

➤ **The Confluence of Elegance and innovation in Fashion**. Explore how Manhattan's fashion scene is a perfect fusion of elegance and innovation. Dive into the evolution of fashion in the city, where classic styles meet cutting-edge trends, and designers continually redefine the boundaries of creativity.

➤ **Personal Expression: Where Elegance Meets Innovation**. Delve into how Manhattan's elite use personal expression as a canvas to blend elegance and innovation. Discuss how this confluence of style, technology, and individuality becomes a powerful means of self-expression in the city that celebrates uniqueness.

➢ **Architectural Marvels: Skyscrapers and Sanctuaries**. Dive into the architectural wonders of Manhattan, from awe-inspiring skyscrapers to tranquil sanctuaries. Explore how these structures embody the city's blend of historical elegance and cutting-edge innovation, each building telling its own story of cultural and aesthetic evolution.

➢ **Culinary Creativity: Dining as an Art Form**. Experience Manhattan's culinary scene, where dining is elevated to an art form. Consider how top chefs in the city fuse traditional flavors with modern techniques to create dishes that are not only a feast for the palate but also a spectacle for the eyes, reflecting Manhattan's ethos of elegance and innovation.

➢ **Tech and Connectivity: Wiring the City of Dreams**. Uncover how Manhattan stays at the forefront of technological advancement, from smart city initiatives to the integration of AI in everyday life. This section highlights how technology enhances the efficiency and luxury that Manhattanites expect, pushing boundaries to create a seamlessly connected urban experience.

➢ **Artistic Influence: The Pulse of the Art World**. Examine Manhattan's significant influence on the global art scene. From iconic museums and galleries to underground art movements, see how the city fosters a unique blend of classic and contemporary art, making it a central hub for artists who embody both the traditional elegance and innovative spirit of Manhattan.

As we conclude this journey into Manhattan's ethos of elegance and innovation, remember that this city doesn't just appreciate beauty on the surface—it thrives on the depth of character, the audacity of ideas, and the pursuit of excellence. Elegance and innovation are not just ideals; they are a way of life, reflected in every facet of Manhattan's vibrant culture.

*Completed Tasks: Elegance and Innovation Activities*

_____
_____
_____
_____
_____
_____
_____
_____
_____
_____
_____
_____
_____
_____
_____
_____
_____
_____
_____
_____
_____
_____
_____
_____
_____
_____
_____

*Inspirational Quote*

YOUR ORDINARY ACTS OF LOVE AND HOPE POINT TO THE EXTRAORDINARY PROMISE THAT EVERY HUMAN LIFE IS OF INESTIMABLE VALUE. — Desmond Tutu

*Action Items: Intentions and Thoughts*

## Action Items: Intentions and Thoughts

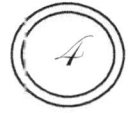

# 4

# Central Park Cleanse: Detoxing Your Skin from City Pollutants

Manhattan, where tales of triumph and tribulations cascade from every rooftop, whispering stories of lives lived large against the backdrop of the ever-pulsating city. Yet, for all its allure and adrenaline, the city's embrace often leaves a smoky imprint—a trace of the relentless hustle and bustle on your pristine skin. In the city that never sleeps, it's not just about conquering the skyline, but about doing so with a radiant glow, a pristine polish, and an untarnished sheen.

Picture this: You're floating down Central Park West, each gaze irresistibly gravitating towards you. It's not the designer tag on your tote that's catching the eye, but the fresh, dewy luminescence of your skin, seemingly untouched by the city's grime. That, my dear, is the Central Park Cleanse, a symbol of purity amidst the urban jungle, a reflection of resilience and rejuvenation.

In this tantalizing episode of The Manhattan Diaries, we delve deep into the alchemy of preserving and reviving your skin from the city's pollutants. From the invigorating morning rituals that kiss away the city's residue to the nocturnal detoxes that lull your skin into a rejuvenating reprieve, you'll learn the coveted secrets of Manhattan's luminous elite.

However, this journey is more than skin-deep. It's an intricate dance with the city's rhythm, a harmonious balance of embracing its vivacity while shielding oneself from its excesses. It's about thriving amidst the towering skyscrapers without letting their shadows diminish your inner glow.

So, step in as we embark on this urban odyssey, embracing the city's fervor while ensuring it doesn't leave its mark. Because, darling, in the theater of Manhattan, every morning is an opportunity for a fresh, radiant debut. The spotlight's on you, and the city's stage is set for your luminous encore.

Welcome to The Manhattan Diaries—where your glow is the only testament needed to your love affair with the city.

## Morning Rituals for a Manhattan Glow

Darling, picture a Manhattan morning—where the city's dreams are still unfolding, and the streets are kissed by the softest light of dawn. In this chapter, we'll uncover the morning rituals that bestow the coveted Manhattan Glow upon the city's elite. It's more than just skincare; it's a dance with the city's essence, a whispered promise of a luminous day ahead. Join me on this journey, as we unveil the secrets to starting your day with the radiance that rivals the Manhattan skyline at sunrise.

- ➤ **The Elixir of Morning Serums**. Explore the enchanting world of morning serums, the elixirs that Manhattan's luminous elite swear by. Learn how these potent concoctions hydrate, rejuvenate, and prepare the skin to face the day with unparalleled luminosity.

- ➤ **The Power of Gentle Cleansing**. Discover the importance of gentle cleansing in the Manhattan morning ritual. It's not just about removing the night's residue; it's about revitalizing the skin, ensuring it's a flawless canvas for the day's adventures.

- ➤ **Sun-Kissed Protections: Shielding Your Skin**. Discuss the significance of sun protection in Manhattan's skincare routine. From UV-blocking creams to protective makeup, understand how the city's dwellers shield their skin from the urban sun's unforgiving embrace.

- ➤ **Awakening the Eyes: Banishing Morning Fatigue**. Uncover the secrets of banishing morning fatigue from the eyes—a crucial element in achieving the Manhattan Glow. Learn about eye creams and treatments that rejuvenate and brighten, ensuring your gaze is as vibrant as the city itself.

➤ **The Art of Exfoliation: Radiance in Every Scrub**. Delve into the art of exfoliation in Manhattan's morning ritual. Explore the gentle yet effective ways Manhattan's elite rid their skin of dullness, revealing a radiant complexion underneath.

➤ **Hydration Beyond Creams: The Magic of Face Mists**. Discover the magic of face mists in Manhattan's skincare routine. Understand how these hydrating spritzes keep the skin refreshed and glowing throughout the day, no matter what the city's demands.

➤ **Morning Massages: The Secret to Skin's Vitality**. Explore the rejuvenating power of morning facial massages. Learn how Manhattan's radiant elite incorporate this tactile ritual to stimulate blood circulation, reduce puffiness, and promote a healthy, youthful complexion.

➤ **Mindful Morning Moments: Incorporating Mindfulness**. Delve into the importance of mindfulness in the Manhattan morning ritual. Consider how taking a moment for self-reflection and gratitude adds an inner glow that radiates throughout the day, embracing the city's vivacity with serenity and grace.

As we conclude our exploration of morning rituals for a Manhattan Glow, remember that here, every day is a fresh canvas, and your skincare routine is the artist's brush. It's not just about looking radiant; it's about feeling the city's energy course through you as you step into the bustling streets. Welcome to The Manhattan Diaries, where each morning is a promise of a luminous day, and your glow becomes a testament to your love affair with this dazzling city.

*Completed Tasks: Facial Glow Rituals Activities*

_____

_____

_____

_____

_____

_____

_____

_____

_____

_____

_____

_____

_____

_____

_____

_____

_____

_____

_____

_____

_____

_____

_____

_____

_____

_____

_____

_____

_____

*Inspirational Quote*

WHAT WE NEED IS MORE PEOPLE WHO SPECIALIZE IN THE IMPOSSIBLE. —
Theodore Roethke

*Action Items: Intentions and Thoughts*

## *Nocturnal Detox: Unwinding Your Skin After Dark*

Picture a Manhattan night—the city that never truly sleeps, where the moonlight dances on skyscraper facades and the streets whisper secrets known only to those who embrace the nocturnal mystique. In this chapter, we uncover the secrets of the Nocturnal Detox, a ritual cherished by Manhattan's luminous elite. It's not just about skincare; it's about unwinding your skin after the dark adventures of the city. Join me as we journey through the night, unveiling the exquisite art of rejuvenation that ensures you wake up with a complexion as luminous as the city's stars.

> ➢ **The Nocturnal Elixir: Overnight Serums and Oils**. Ah, the Nocturnal Elixir—the secret potion of Manhattan's radiant elite. These overnight serums and oils work their magic while you dream, rejuvenating your skin and ensuring you wake up looking as glamorous as a Manhattan star.

> ➢ **Nightly Cleansing Ritual: Washing Away the Day**. You can't conquer the night without a proper cleansing ritual. It's not just about removing makeup; it's about shedding the day's stress and letting your skin breathe freely as you prepare for a night of beauty sleep.

> ➢ **Beauty Sleep Essentials: Silk Pillowcases and Sleep Masks**. Sleeping like a Manhattan elite means resting your head on silk pillowcases and donning luxurious sleep masks. These essentials not only pamper you but also enhance your skin's rejuvenation process. Wake up feeling like royalty.

> ➢ **The Magic of Overnight Masks: Skin's Nighttime Replenishment**. Overnight masks—the skincare equivalent of Cinderella's glass slipper. These magical masks provide your skin with the deep nourishment it craves while you slumber, ensuring you wake up with a glow that rivals the city's nightlife.

- ➤ **Luxurious Nighttime Rituals**. Embrace the allure of luxurious nighttime rituals—indulge in scented candles, calming music, and the soothing touch of silk sheets. Creating an ambiance of opulence enhances your skin's relaxation and rejuvenation.

- ➤ **Hydration Overnight: Sleep with a Hydrating Mist**. Let's talk about the beauty of hydration overnight. Spritzing your face with a hydrating mist before bed keeps your skin refreshed and plump, ensuring you wake up with that coveted morning glow.

- ➤ **Silent Night's Dream: Mindfulness Before Sleep**. Unwind your mind with a touch of mindfulness before drifting into slumber. Just a few moments of tranquility and gratitude can enhance your sleep quality, leaving you refreshed and radiant in the morning.

- ➤ **Rejuvenating Night Creams: Enhancing Skin's Elasticity**. Delve into the benefits of rejuvenating night creams that work to enhance your skin's elasticity and firmness as you sleep. These creams are enriched with peptides and antioxidants, helping to repair daily environmental damage and improve skin texture for a youthful, revitalized appearance by morning.

- ➤ **Essential Oils for Serenity**. Infuse your evening routine with essential oils known for their calming properties. A few drops of lavender or chamomile oil can transform your bedroom into a sanctuary for rest, enhancing your skin's ability to regenerate overnight.

As we conclude our exploration of the Nocturnal Detox, remember that Manhattan nights are as much a part of your skincare routine as the mornings. It's about allowing your skin to unwind, rejuvenate, and embrace the city's nocturnal energy. Welcome to The Manhattan Diaries, where each night is an opportunity for your skin to experience the enchanting Nocturnal Detox, ensuring you rise with a complexion that rivals the moonlit skyline.

## Completed Tasks: Skin After Dark Activities

_____

_____

_____

_____

_____

_____

_____

_____

_____

_____

_____

_____

_____

_____

_____

_____

_____

_____

_____

_____

_____

_____

_____

_____

_____

_____

_____

_____

_____

_____

_____

_____

_____

_Inspirational Quote_

FOR A GALLANT SPIRIT THERE CAN NEVER BE DEFEAT. — Wallis Simpson

*Action Items: Intentions and Thoughts*

*Shielding Your Glow: Protecting Skin from City Pollutants*

Ah, Manhattan, where the streets are paved with dreams and every corner tells a story of ambition and allure. But, my darlings, amidst the city's splendor lies a hidden challenge—protecting your radiant glow from the relentless embrace of urban pollutants. In this captivating chapter, we dive into the art of Shielding Your Glow, a secret closely guarded by Manhattan's luminous elite. It's not just about skincare; it's about crafting a shield that lets you conquer the city while preserving your flawless charm. Join me as we explore the secrets of safeguarding your glow in the city that never sleeps.

> ➢ **Urban Armor: The Power of Antioxidants**. Let's talk about urban armor, my loves. Antioxidants are your best friends in the Manhattan battle against pollutants. They're like a shield, protecting your skin from the city's harsh elements and keeping your complexion as vibrant as the city lights.

> ➢ **Detoxifying Cleansers: Washing Away the City's Grime**. Oh, but the city's grime can be relentless. Detoxifying cleansers are your go-to for purging the day's impurities, leaving your skin refreshed and ready to face another Manhattan adventure.

> ➢ **City-Proof Sunscreens: Your Daily Defense**. And of course, we can't forget about sunscreen, especially one that's city-proof. It's like a chic accessory for your skin, shielding you from the sun's rays and the city's smog with equal grace.

> ➢ **Revival Elixirs: Nightly Rejuvenation**. But the nighttime is when the magic happens, my darlings. Revival elixirs are the secret to nightly rejuvenation, ensuring you wake up looking as flawless as you did when you entered the city's whirlwind.

> ➢ **Mist on the Go: Refreshing Face Sprays**. For those moments on the bustling Manhattan streets, keep refreshing face sprays close at

hand. A quick spritz revitalizes your skin and spirit, making the city's chaos feel like a breeze.

➢ **Detox Masks: Weekly Purification Rituals**. Don't forget to indulge in detox masks as part of your weekly purification ritual. They're like a mini getaway for your skin, flushing out impurities and leaving you feeling reborn, ready to take on the city once more.

➢ **Glow-Boosting Serums: The City's Best-Kept Secret**. Glow-boosting serums are the city's best-kept secret, my dears. These little wonders not only protect your skin from pollutants but also enhance your natural radiance, ensuring you shine amidst the Manhattan skyline.

➢ **Hydration from Within: Sip on Skin-Boosting Elixirs**. And, lovelies, don't forget that hydration from within is just as crucial. Sip on skin-boosting elixirs like collagen-infused beverages or herbal teas to keep your skin plump and radiant, even in the city's hustle and bustle.

➢ **Barrier-Enhancing Moisturizers: Daily Skin Fortification**. Round out your protective regimen with barrier-enhancing moisturizers. These daily essentials fortify your skin's natural defenses, sealing in hydration and nutrients while keeping environmental pollutants out, ensuring your skin remains resilient against the urban elements.

As we wrap up our exploration of Shielding Your Glow, remember that Manhattan is a love affair that requires a little protection. Your skincare routine becomes the armor that allows you to embrace the city's vibrancy while preserving your signature radiance. Welcome to The Manhattan Diaries, where your glow is as resilient as your spirit, and every day in the city is a new chapter waiting to be written.

## Completed Tasks: Shielding Your Glow Activities

_____
_____
_____
_____
_____
_____
_____
_____
_____
_____
_____
_____
_____
_____
_____
_____
_____
_____
_____
_____
_____
_____
_____
_____
_____
_____
_____
_____

_Inspirational Quote_

THERE ARE GLIMPSES OF HEAVEN TO US IN EVERY ACT, OR THOUGHT, OR WORD THAT RAISES US ABOVE OURSELVES. — Robert Quillen

*Action Items: Intentions and Thoughts*

## *Beyond Skincare: The Mind-Body Connection*

Darlings, in the dazzling labyrinth of Manhattan, where ambition and allure reign supreme, we're about to embark on a journey that goes beyond skincare. Yes, you heard me right—it's time to explore the Mind-Body Connection, the secret to radiance that's as much about inner harmony as it is about flawless skin. In this enchanting chapter, we'll uncover how Manhattan's luminous elite blend the art of self-care with the city's vibrant spirit. It's a symphony of balance, my loves, where the soul's radiance complements the glow on your skin. Join me as we delve into the secrets of a harmonious life in the city that never sleeps.

➢ **Meditation and Morning Zen: Finding Inner Calm**. Let's begin with meditation, darlings—the morning zen that sets the tone for your day. Manhattan's radiant souls know that finding inner calm amidst the city's chaos is the key to maintaining their signature glow.

➢ **Soulful Nutrition: Eating for Radiance**. Next, we dive into soulful nutrition because beauty starts from within. Manhattan's elite indulge in nourishing their bodies with foods that not only taste divine but also promote a radiant complexion.

➢ **Elevating Fitness Routines: Sculpting a Vibrant Spirt**. Fitness routines in Manhattan are not just about sweating it out; they're about sculpting a vibrant spirit. From boutique fitness studios to rooftop yoga sessions, the city's luminous souls ensure their bodies are as dynamic as their lives.

➢ **Nightly Rituals for Inner Peace: Sleep as a Beauty Elixir**. And as we wind down the day, let's talk about nightly rituals for inner peace. Manhattan's elite understand that sleep is the ultimate beauty elixir, and they create bedtime routines that guarantee a night of rejuvenating rest.

➢ **Cultivating Inner Glow: Stress Management Strategies.** Stress management is an art that Manhattan's luminous souls have mastered. They incorporate strategies like mindfulness, deep breathing, and occasional spa escapes to keep their inner glow undiminished by the city's demands.

➢ **Hydration Elevation: Sip on Skin-Boosting Infusions.** Hydration isn't just about skincare; it's about sipping on skin-boosting infusions throughout the day. Manhattan's elite opt for herbal teas, collagen-infused waters, and vitamin-rich concoctions to keep their bodies and skin hydrated.

➢ **Mindful Escapes: Weekend Retreats and Getaways.** Weekend retreats and getaways are an essential part of Manhattan's elite lifestyle. These mindful escapes allow them to recharge, rejuvenate, and come back to the city with renewed energy and radiance.

➢ **Community Connection: Cultivating Meaningful Relationships.** Last but certainly not least, cultivating meaningful relationships and a sense of community is vital. Manhattan's luminous souls understand the importance of surrounding themselves with positive influences, which adds to their inner and outer glow.

As we conclude our journey through the Mind-Body Connection in The Manhattan Diaries, remember that Manhattan's magic isn't just visible—it's deeply felt. Your inner glow, fueled by both mind and spirit, shines as brightly as any city light. Here, every day is a celebration of your vibrant essence, a testament to the profound connection between your well-being and the city's energetic pulse. Embrace this union of mind, body, and spirit, and let Manhattan refine your radiance, making every moment a tribute to your personal growth and inner beauty.

# URBAN ELIXIR

## Completed Tasks: Mind-Body Connection Activities

# CENTRAL PARK CLEANSE

*Action Items: Intentions and Thoughts*

## *Embracing Manhattan's Rhythm*

Darlings, welcome to the heart of Manhattan—the dazzling, relentless urban jungle where every heartbeat echoes with ambition and allure. Today, we're diving into the art of Embracing Manhattan's Rhythm, a dance that balances the city's vivacity with the radiance of your inner glow. In this enthralling chapter, we'll uncover how Manhattan's luminous elite synchronize their lives with the city's vibrant pulse. It's a delicate harmony, my loves, where the urban rhythm becomes the backdrop for your radiant journey. Join me as we explore the secrets of embracing the city's fervor while ensuring your inner light shines even brighter.

> ➢ **Cityscape Inspiration: Drawing from Urban Energy**. Picture it, my darlings—Manhattan's skyline as your muse. The city's relentless energy, its towering skyscrapers, the rush of the streets—it's all a part of your creative canvas. Let it inspire you, drive you, and infuse your life with an electric vibrancy that matches the city's own heartbeat.

> ➢ **Urban Nature Retreats: Finding Serenity Amidst Skyscrapers**. Now, let's talk about urban nature retreats—a haven amidst the concrete jungle. Imagine strolling through Central Park, with the city's hustle and bustle mere whispers in the distance. These moments of serenity are like a balm for your soul, providing a much-needed respite from Manhattan's relentless pace.

> ➢ **Sensory Exploration: Savoring Manhattan's Culinary Delights**. Ah, the culinary delights of Manhattan! Think of it as a symphony for your taste buds. Explore the city's diverse food scene, from gourmet eateries to hidden gems, savoring every flavor as if it were a work of art; it's a sensory journey that elevates your spirit.

> ➢ **Cultural Immersion: Nurturing the Soul with Arts and Theater**. And, my loves, don't forget the arts and theater. Manhattan's cultural scene is a treasure trove waiting to be discovered. Attend Broadway

shows, explore art exhibitions, and immerse yourself in performances that ignite your passion for creativity. It's soul-nourishing, like a love affair with the city itself.

➢ **Cityscape Workspaces: Elevating Productivity in the Heart of Manhattan**. Imagine, darling, your workspace in the heart of Manhattan's cityscape. Manhattan's elite know that a well-designed workspace can boost productivity while keeping you connected to the city's vibrant energy.

➢ **Midday Mindfulness: Taking Short Breaks for Inner Rejuvenation**. Midday mindfulness breaks are a must. In the midst of Manhattan's hustle, take a few moments for inner rejuvenation. Close your eyes, breathe deeply, and let the city's energy recharge your spirit.

➢ **Exploring Hidden Gems: Unearthing Manhattan's Best-Kept Secrets**. Unearth the city's best-kept secrets—hidden gems that only the true Manhattan connoisseurs know about. From speakeasy bars to boutique shops, these discoveries add a touch of exclusivity to your urban experience.

➢ **Fashion Forward: Embracing Manhattan's Style Evolution**. And, of course, let's not forget fashion. Embrace Manhattan's style evolution, my loves. The city's fashion scene is ever-evolving, and being at the forefront of trends is a testament to your commitment to Manhattan's allure.

As we wrap up our exploration of Embracing Manhattan's Rhythm, remember that the city is your muse, your sanctuary, your inspiration. The urban vibrancy and your inner glow are intertwined, creating a symphony of life that's uniquely Manhattan. Welcome to The Manhattan Diaries, where every day is a chance to dance to the city's rhythm and let your radiance shine amidst its dazzling lights.

# Completed Tasks: City Rhythm Activities

---

_Inspirational Quote_

REACH FOR THE STARS. — Christa McAuliffe

# CENTRAL PARK CLEANSE

*Action Items: Intentions and Thoughts*

*Action Items: Intentions and Thoughts*

_____

_____

_____

_____

_____

_____

_____

_____

_____

_____

_____

_____

_____

_____

_____

_____

_____

_____

_____

_____

_____

_____

_____

_____

_____

_____

_____

_____

_____

_____

_____

_____

# Broadway's Barrier Boost: Strengthening Defenses Against Urban Elements

Manhattan—a radiant beacon, pulsating with dreams, dramas, and an electrifying energy that surges through its veins. In this city where the spotlight is relentless, the backdrop becomes as essential as the performance. And just as every Broadway star needs a robust defense against the spotlight's heat, your skin yearns for a barrier against the city's unyielding elements.

Envision it now: there you are, serenely strolling down Broadway, the theaters' luminous marquees paling in the comparison to your radiant glow. It's not your ensemble that's commanding attention, but the radiant barrier that seems to envelope you—a shield, both subtle and strong, against Manhattan's demanding tempo. That, darling, is the Broadway Barrier Boost, an emblem of resilience, an armor of elegance.

In this thrilling installment of The Manhattan Diaries, you'll draw back the curtain on the secrets of the city's most protected. From the meticulously layered elixirs that fortify and nourish to the spritzes that set the safeguard, you'll unravel the regimes of those who face the city's trials head-on, yet emerge untouched, untarnished.

But this isn't solely a superficial sojourn. This is about syncing with the city's heartbeat, aligning your defenses with its challenges, and choreographing a routine that not only endures but thrives. It's about understanding that while Manhattan might test you, with the right armor, its challenges become your triumphs.

So, accompany me on this urban escapade, as we tune into the melodies of the city absorbing its rhythms while deftly deflecting its blows. For in the grand theater of Manhattan, every day is your opening night, and the world is eagerly awaiting your encore. Welcome to The Manhattan Diaries—where your resilience becomes as legendary as the city's tales.

## *Broadway's Beauty Armor: Secrets of Skin Protection*

Darlings, welcome to a chapter that's all about indulging in the secrets of Broadway's Beauty Armor. In the dazzling world of Manhattan, where every day feels like a performance, your skin needs a shield against the city's unyielding elements. Picture it: luminous souls strolling down Broadway, their skin protected by an elegant, invisible armor. In The Manhattan Diaries, we'll uncover the meticulously crafted regimes, elixirs, and spritzes that keep them radiant amidst the chaos. It's not just about beauty; it's about resilience.

> ➤ **The First Act: Layered Elixirs for Ultimate Protection**. Our first act reveals the magic of layered elixirs. Manhattan's elite understand the importance of a well-crafted skincare routine. They layer potions and serums, creating a fortress that shields their skin from the city's harsh elements. It's a secret recipe that keeps their glow intact.

> ➤ **The Second Act: Spritzing the Safeguard**. Next, we enter the second act, where spritzing takes center stage. Manhattan's luminous souls have a knack for choosing the perfect spritzes. These refreshing mists set the safeguard, creating a protective veil that keeps the city at bay. It's a ritual that adds elegance to their daily routine.

> ➤ **The Third Act: Resilience Amidst the Chaos**. In our third act, we explore resilience amidst the chaos. Manhattan's beauty warriors know that it's not just about looking flawless; it's about being resilient. They align their defenses with the city's challenges, turning every obstacle into an opportunity for triumph.

> ➤ **Curtain Call: Broadway's Beauty Unveiled**. As we reach the curtain call, remember that beauty in Manhattan isn't just a facade—it's a testament to inner strength. In The Manhattan Diaries, we celebrate the city's luminous souls and their radiant armor. Every day in this grand theater is a chance for your resilience to shine as bright

as the city itself. Welcome, darlings, to a world where beauty and strength go hand in hand.

➢ **The Fourth Act: Skincare Elixirs with Manhattan Flair**. In our fourth act, we delve deeper into skincare elixirs with a Manhattan flair. Discover the elixirs that Manhattan's beauty connoisseurs swear by—products infused with a touch of magic, specially crafted to combat the city's challenges while keeping your skin luminous.

➢ **The Fifth Act: Daily Rituals for a Resilient Glow**. This act focuses on the daily rituals that create a resilient glow. Manhattan's radiant elite have mastered the art of incorporating skincare into their bustling lives. We'll unveil their daily routines, offering insights into how you can effortlessly maintain your barrier against the city's elements.

➢ **The Sixth Act: Age-Defying Secrets of Manhattan's Icons**. In our sixth act, we'll uncover age-defying secrets. Manhattan's icons have mastered the art of maintaining youthful skin, even amidst the city's relentless pace. Discover the potions and elixirs they rely on to keep those fine lines and wrinkles at bay.

➢ **The Grand Finale: The Power of Confidence and Resilience**. As we reach the grand finale, remember that it's not just about products; it's about the power of confidence and resilience. Manhattan's luminous souls wear their armor with grace, and it's their inner strength that truly sets them apart.

As we wrap up our exploration of Embracing Manhattan's Rhythm, remember that the city is your muse, your sanctuary, your inspiration. The urban vibrancy and your inner glow are intertwined, creating a symphony of life that's uniquely Manhattan. Welcome to The Manhattan Diaries, where every day is a chance to dance to the city's rhythm and let your radiance shine amidst its dazzling lights.

## Completed Tasks: Beauty Armor Activities

_Inspirational Quote_

ONE TODAY IS WORTH TWO TOMORROWS. — Benjamin Franklin

*Action Items: Intentions and Thoughts*

*Defying Urban Elements: Nourishing and Fortifying Your Skin*

Darlings, let's embark on a journey that's all about defying urban elements and nourishing your skin. In the heart of Manhattan's relentless energy, your skin deserves the utmost care and fortification. Picture it: you, gracefully navigating the city's chaos, your skin radiating a luminous glow that defies the harsh urban elements. In The Manhattan Diaries, we'll dive into the art of nurturing and fortifying your skin, revealing the secrets of Manhattan's luminous elite.

➢ **The First Step: A Ritual of Hydration and Moisture**. Our first step is all about hydration and moisture. Manhattan's radiant souls understand that the city's pace can leave skin parched. They have a ritual that includes rich hydrating products, keeping their skin supple and resilient against the urban elements.

➢ **The Second Step: The Power of Antioxidants**. Next, we uncover the power of antioxidants. Manhattan's luminous icons swear by products rich in antioxidants, which shield their skin from the pollution and stress of city life. These elixirs act as a protective barrier, preserving their youthful radiance.

➢ **The Third Step: Essential Vitamins for Skin Resilience**. In our third step, we delve into essential vitamins for skin resilience. Manhattan's beauty connoisseurs know that nourishing the skin from within is essential. We'll explore the vitamins and nutrients they incorporate into their routines, giving their skin the strength to endure.

➢ **Curtain Call: The Resilient Beauty of Manhattan**. As we reach our curtain call, remember that beauty in Manhattan isn't just about looking flawless—it's about being resilient. In The Manhattan Diaries, we celebrate the city's luminous souls and their dedication to nurturing and fortifying their skin. Your journey here isn't just about skincare; it's about embracing the city's challenges and emerging as a resilient star. Welcome, darlings, to a world where your beauty defies the urban elements with elegance and grace.

- ➤ **The Fourth Step: Restorative Nighttime Rituals**. In our fourth step, we explore the importance of restorative nighttime rituals. Manhattan's luminous elite have perfected their skincare routines, even as they sleep. Discover the luxurious products and techniques they use to rejuvenate their skin during the night, ensuring it remains resilient and youthful.

- ➤ **The Fifth Step: Balancing Act for City-Dwelling Skin**. This step is all about finding the perfect balance for city-dwelling skin. Manhattan's radiant souls understand that skincare is a delicate dance. Uncover their secrets for achieving the ideal equilibrium between hydration, protection, and nourishment, ensuring their skin stays resilient in the face of urban challenges.

- ➤ **The Sixth Step: Serums and Elixirs for Urban Warriors**. In our sixth step, we delve into the serums and elixirs favored by Manhattan's urban warriors. These products are specifically crafted to combat the effects of city life. Discover the luxurious concoctions that form the foundation of their skincare arsenals, helping them maintain their luminous glow.

As we approach the grand finale, remember that it's not just about products; it's about the radiant confidence that comes from caring for your skin in the urban jungle. Manhattan's luminous souls know that resilient skin is a testament to inner strength. Your journey in The Manhattan Diaries isn't just about skincare; it's about embracing the city's challenges with elegance and grace, emerging as a radiant star in your own right.

## Completed Tasks: Nourishing and Fortifying Activities

_____

_____

_____

_____

_____

_____

_____

_____

_____

_____

_____

_____

_____

_____

_____

_____

_____

_____

_____

_____

_____

_____

_____

_____

_____

_____

_____

_____

*Inspirational Quote*

WE CAN CHANGE OUR LIVES. WE CAN DO, HAVE, AND BE EXACTLY WHAT WE WISH. — Tony Robbins

# BROADWAY'S BARRIER BOOST

*Action Items: Intentions and Thoughts*

95

## *Syncing with Manhattan's Rhythm*

Darlings, welcome to a chapter that's all about syncing with Manhattan's rhythm and aligning your defenses with its challenges. In this city of relentless energy, it's not just about conquering the streets—it's about thriving amidst the chaos. Picture it: you, gracefully navigating the bustling avenues, your skin a radiant shield against the city's demands. In The Manhattan Diaries, we'll explore the art of harmonizing with Manhattan's rhythm, revealing the secrets of those who not only endure but flourish in this urban jungle.

- ➢ **The First Beat: Understanding Manhattan's Unique Demands**. Our first beat is about understanding Manhattan's unique demands. It's essential to recognize the city's pace and the toll it can take on your skin. Manhattan's luminous elite are well-versed in these challenges and have tailored their skincare routines accordingly.

- ➢ **The Second Beat: Daytime Defense Strategies**. Next, we delve into daytime defense strategies. Manhattan's beauty connoisseurs have devised meticulous plans for protecting their skin during the day. From SPF-infused products to urban shield elixirs, they ensure their skin remains resilient in the face of pollution and stress.

- ➢ **The Third Beat: Nighttime Rejuvenation Rituals**. In our third beat, explore nighttime rejuvenation rituals. Manhattan's radiant souls understand the importance of nighttime recovery. Unveil their indulgent practices, including restorative masks and serums that help their skin heal and regenerate while they sleep.

- ➢ **Curtain Call: Thriving in Manhattan's Grand Theater**. As we approach the curtain call, remember that it's not just about skincare—it's about syncing with the city's pulse and emerging stronger. In The Manhattan Diaries, we celebrate those who thrive in Manhattan's grand theater. Your journey here isn't just about looking radiant; it's about aligning your defenses with the city's challenges, mastering its rhythm, and becoming a star in your own right. Welcome, darlings, to a world where your beauty harmonizes with the city's heartbeat.

➢ **The Fourth Beat: Tailoring Your Skincare Arsenal**. In our fourth beat, we emphasize the importance of tailoring your skincare arsenal. Manhattan's luminous elite understand that not all skincare products are created equal. Discover how they curate their collection of potions and elixirs to address their specific needs and adapt to the city's ever-changing environment.

➢ **The Fifth Beat: Mindful Urban Living**. This beat focuses on mindful urban living. Manhattan's radiant souls know that skincare isn't just about external products—it's about a holistic approach to well-being. Explore their practices of mindfulness, stress management, and urban living that contribute to their overall resilience and glow.

➢ **The Sixth Beat: The Art of Inner Radiance**. In our sixth beat, we delve into the art of inner radiance. Manhattan's luminous icons radiate not just because of their skincare routines but because of their inner strength and confidence. Discover the secrets to cultivating that inner glow that sets you apart in the city that never sleeps.

As we reach the grand finale, remember that it's not just about products; it's about thriving amidst Manhattan's symphony. Manhattan's luminous souls have mastered the art of synchronizing with the city's rhythm, aligning their defenses with its challenges, and emerging as radiant stars. Your journey in The Manhattan Diaries isn't just about skincare; it's about becoming a part of the city's vibrant symphony, where your glow shines alongside the city's brilliance.

## Completed Tasks: Syncing with Rhythm Activities

_____
_____
_____
_____
_____
_____
_____
_____
_____
_____
_____
_____
_____
_____
_____
_____
_____
_____
_____
_____
_____
_____
_____
_____
_____

_Inspirational Quote_

GREAT HOPES MAKE GREAT MEN. —— Thomas Fuller

*Action Items: Intentions and Thoughts*

## *Broadway's Resilience Rituals*

Darlings, it's time to uncover the resilience rituals of Broadway—the grand theater of Manhattan. In this city of dreams and drama, where every spotlight is relentless, your skin needs a routine that can withstand the stage's intensity. Picture it: you, center stage on Broadway, your skin as radiant as the marquee lights, stealing the show. In The Manhattan Diaries, we'll explore the secrets of Broadway's resilient stars, those who understand that their skin must be as unyielding as their performances.

> ➤ **The First Act: Preparing the Canvas—Skincare as a Ritual**. Our first act is all about preparing the canvas. Skincare isn't just a routine; it's a ritual. Manhattan's luminous elite treat their skincare routines like a performance, starting with gentle cleansing and exfoliation to create the perfect canvas for their radiant glow.

> ➤ **The Second Act: Show-Stopping Ingredients—Luxury in a Bottle**. Next, dive into the show-stopping ingredients that Manhattan's stars swear by. From luxurious serums infused with rare extracts to moisturizers that deliver instant luminosity, discover the elixirs that give their skin a red carpet-worthy radiance.

> ➤ **The Third Act: On-Stage Glow—Makeup as an Enhancement**. In our third act, explore the on-stage glow achieved through makeup. Manhattan's radiant souls know that makeup is an enhancement, not a mask. Unveil their makeup tricks and techniques that amplify their natural beauty, ensuring they shine even under the spotlight.

> ➤ **Curtain Call: Resilience as a Star Quality**. As we approach the curtain call, remember that resilience is a star quality. In The Manhattan Diaries, we celebrate those who understand that their skincare and beauty routines must be as unwavering as their performances. Your journey here isn't just about looking glamorous;

it's about embracing the stage's intensity with grace and confidence, becoming a star in your own right. Welcome, darlings, to a world where your resilience shines as brightly as the Broadway lights.

➤ **The Fourth Act: Nourishing the Skin's Vital Role**. In our fourth act, we emphasize the vital role of nourishing the skin. Manhattan's luminous elite understand that well-nourished skin is the foundation of radiance. Discover the luxurious treatments and masks they indulge in to keep their skin healthy, vibrant, and ready for the spotlight.

➤ **The Fifth Act: Post-Performance Recovery**. This act focuses on post-performance recovery. After the curtain falls, it's essential to give your skin the care it deserves. Explore the pampering routines and products that Manhattan's radiant stars use to unwind and rejuvenate, ensuring their skin remains resilient for future performances.

➤ **The Sixth Act: Beauty from Within—Wellness and Nutrition**. In our sixth act, we delve into the concept of beauty from within. Manhattan's luminous icons know that skincare is not just external—it's about wellness and nutrition. Discover their secrets for maintaining a healthy lifestyle that complements their skincare routines, ensuring their inner radiance shines through.

As we reach the grand finale, remember that it's not just about products; it's about resilience as a lifestyle. Manhattan's radiant souls have mastered the art of embracing the stage's intensity while maintaining their skin's strength and vitality. Your journey in The Manhattan Diaries isn't just about skincare; it's about becoming a star on the grand theater of Manhattan, where your resilience shines as brightly as the Broadway lights.

# URBAN ELIXIR

*Completed Tasks: Resilience Rituals Activities*

_____
_____
_____
_____
_____
_____
_____
_____
_____
_____
_____
_____
_____
_____
_____
_____
_____
_____
_____
_____
_____
_____
_____
_____
_____
_____
_____
_____

*Inspirational Quote*

TO THE MIND THAT IS STILL, THE WHOLE UNIVERSE SURRENDERS. — Lao Tzu

# BROADWAY'S BARRIER BOOST

*Action Items: Intentions and Thoughts*

*Action Items: Intentions and Thoughts*

# 6

# Fifth Avenue Facials:
## The Elite's Go-To for Monthly Skin Refinement

Manhattan—the urban jungle where legends are made, and legacies are forged. Here, amidst the crescendo of car horns and the symphony of street chatter, every move is scrutinized, every gesture examined. And in this relentless city, it's not just about claiming your space; it's about doing so with a radiant flourish and a flawless finish.

Visualize this: As you saunter down the iconic Fifth Avenue, gazes lock onto you, captivated, not by the glint of your accessories, but the luminous canvas of your face. That glow, dear reader, is the Fifth Avenue Facial Effect—an emblem of opulence, a testament to the city's elite's commitment to perfecting their visage.

In this tantalizing entry of The Manhattan Diaries, we delve deep into the clandestine chambers of Manhattan's skin care sanctuaries. From the meticulously crafted treatments that harness ancient wisdom and modern marvels to the whispered secrets of the crème de la crème, you're about to gain access to a world where refinement is a ritual, not a luxury.

But understand, this isn't just about surface splendor. It's about harmonizing with the city's dynamic pulse, about wearing your stories, your ambitions, your dreams on the most intimate canvas—your skin. It's about standing tall amid the steel sentinels, reflecting their grandeur and the soft allure of the parks below.

So, let's embark on this skin-deep soiree, attuning to the undercurrents of the city, absorbing its essence, and exuding its elegance. Because in Manhattan, every glance in your direction is an unspoken accolade, a nod to your commitment to perfection. Welcome to The Manhattan Diaries—where your radiance rivals the city lights.

## *The Secret Sanctuaries*

In the bustling heart of Manhattan, where the city's pulse beats loudest, there exist hidden oases of tranquility and luxury—the secret sanctuaries of the city's elite. These exclusive skincare havens, tucked away behind unassuming facades or perched atop glittering skyscrapers, are where the beauty rituals of Manhattan's most discerning denizens unfold. These are not mere spas; they are the temples of rejuvenation, where the city's high and mighty retreat to refine and perfect their skin, away from the prying eyes and relentless pace of city life.

➢ **The Decreet Doorways: Entrances to Elegance**. Each sanctuary begins with a discreet entrance, often hidden in plain sight, offering an escape from the urban frenzy into a world of serene luxury.

➢ **The Personalized Chambers: Bespoke Beauty Abodes**. Inside, personalized chambers await, each tailored to provide an intimate and luxurious experience. These spaces are designed for comfort, privacy, and complete immersion in the art of skincare.

➢ **The Elite Clientele: Who's Who of Manhattan**. These sanctuaries cater to a clientele that's as exclusive as the treatments they offer. A roster of Manhattan's who's who, from celebrities to business moguls, frequent these spots, each seeking their unique path to skin perfection.

➢ **The Signature Treatments: Coveted Skincare Rituals**. The treatments offered are as coveted as the sanctuaries themselves. From age-defying therapies to revolutionary skin-enhancing techniques, each ritual is a blend of science, art, and luxury.

➢ **The Aromatic Ambiance**. Picture this: as you step further into these sanctuaries, a symphony of subtle scents greets you. Each fragrance is carefully curated to calm the mind and elevate the spirit, setting the stage for a skincare journey that's as much about inner serenity as outer beauty.

- ➤ **The Mastery of Technique**. In these chambers, skilled artisans of skincare work their magic. With every precise touch and expert stroke, they not only tend to your skin but also to your soul. Their techniques are not just procedures; they are performances, where mastery meets intuition in a dance of rejuvenation.

- ➤ **The Whispered Recommendations**. Listen closely, and you might catch the soft murmur of recommendations being passed among Manhattan's elite. It's in these whispers that the secrets of the next big skincare trend are shared, a clandestine exchange of the city's most guarded beauty revelations.

- ➤ **The Lasting Impressions**. And when you finally step back onto the bustling streets, you carry with you more than just a glowing visage. You leave with an impression, an indelible mark of an experience that transcends the ordinary. It's a feeling, a memory, a promise of return to these hidden havens of beauty and luxury.

- ➤ **The Symphony of Service: Exceptional Care and Attentiveness**. Beyond the aesthetic enhancements and skincare miracles, what truly distinguishes these sanctuaries is the exceptional level of service, ensuring that every visit is as memorable for the service as it is for the results.

In the heart of Manhattan, these secret sanctuaries stand as bastions of beauty and refinement. They are more than just spas; they are the sacred spaces where the city's elite come to pause, rejuvenate, and transform. Each visit is an affirmation of their status, a testament to their dedication to maintaining not just their skin but the very essence of their persona. In these hallowed halls, beauty is not just preserved; it is elevated to an art form, reflecting the sophistication and grandeur of the city itself.

*Completed Tasks: Secret Sanctuaries Activities*

_____

_____

_____

_____

_____

_____

_____

_____

_____

_____

_____

_____

_____

_____

_____

_____

_____

_____

_____

_____

_____

_____

_____

_____

*Inspirational Quote*

THE AUTHENTIC SELF IS THE SOUL MADE VISIBLE. — Sarah Ban Breathnach

*Action Items: Intentions and Thoughts*

*The Fusion of Ancient and Modern*

In the heart of Manhattan's buzzing streets lies a secret whispered among the beauty elite: the fusion of ancient wisdom and modern marvels in the realm of skincare. Here, in the city that's always ahead, the most cherished beauty sanctuaries are blending the mystique of ancient rituals with the dazzle of modern science. This fusion is not just a trend; it's a testimony to Manhattan's love affair with both its storied past and its pulsating present. It's where time-honored traditions meet the pace of the New York minute, creating a skincare experience that's as rich in history as it is in innovation.

➢ **The Herbal Alchemy: Nature's Best Kept Secrets**. Envision potions and lotions steeped in herbal wisdom, passed down through generations. These ancient recipes, infused with modern techniques, become elixirs that soothe, rejuvenate, and restore, much like the city itself—ever-evolving yet deeply rooted.

➢ **The Mineral Miracles: From Earth's Depths to Skyscraper Heights**. Minerals, drawn from the earth's depths, find their way into the jars and bottles of Manhattan's high-rises. Mined from distant lands, these minerals are transformed through cutting-edge processes into skincare gold, marrying the old with the new in a luxurious embrace.

➢ **The Acupressure Artistry: Ancient Touch, Modern Grace**. The timeless art of acupressure, reimagined through the lens of contemporary science, brings a touch of ancient healing to the modern spa experience. Each press and release is a nod to ancestral knowledge, tailored for today's skincare aficionado.

➢ **The Botanical Blends: Centuries of Wisdom in a Jar**. Imagine botanicals that have graced ancient beauty rituals, now blended with modern-day bioactive compounds. This fusion creates a symphony of ingredients, each singing in harmony with Manhattan's rhythm.

➤ **The Aromatic Infusion: Scented Whispers From the Past**. Delight in aromatic infusions that hark back to ancient times. These scents, once the secrets of old-world apothecaries, are now enhanced with modern fragrance technology, enveloping Manhattan's elite in a sensory experience that is both timeless and contemporary.

➤ **The Thermal Therapies: Healing Heat Meets Innovative Techniques**. Meet the transformative power of thermal therapies, rooted in ancient bathing rituals, now reimagined with state-of-the-art temperature control. It's a fusion where the comforting warmth of tradition meets the precision of modern science.

➤ **The Crystal Contours: Gemstones with a Modern Twist**. Embrace the mystical allure of crystal contouring, an ancient practice that used gemstones for rejuvenation, now amplified with the latest in skincare tools. In these modern sanctuaries, crystals glide over skin, merging the earth's energies with the innovations of today.

➤ **The Holistic Harmonization: Balancing Body and Mind**. Experience the holistic approach of integrating body and mind wellness, a concept as ancient as civilization itself, now approached with contemporary techniques. It's a harmonious blend that addresses not just skin, but the overall well-being.

In this fusion of ancient and modern, Manhattan's skincare scene becomes a tapestry of time, woven with threads of bygone eras and contemporary wonders. It's a dance of beauty rituals that transcends time, where each step is a celebration of enduring wisdom and forward-thinking innovation. For the Manhattanite who indulges in this fusion, it's more than a skincare routine; it's a journey through ages, a ritual that honors the past while embracing the future. In the city that never sleeps, these beauty rituals are a reminder that while Manhattan races ahead, it always keeps one eye lovingly on the past.

## Completed Tasks: Ancient with Modern Activities

_____
_____
_____
_____
_____
_____
_____
_____
_____
_____
_____
_____
_____
_____
_____
_____
_____
_____
_____
_____
_____
_____
_____
_____
_____
_____

*Inspirational Quote*

FAITH IS LOVE TAKING THE FORM OF ASPIRATION. — William Ellery Channing

*Action Items: Intentions and Thoughts*

*The Tailored Experience*

In the heart of Manhattan, where individuality reigns supreme and every desire is just a whisper away, there lies the allure of the Tailored Experience in skincare. This isn't your run-of-the-mill facial; it's a journey of customization, where each treatment is as unique as the storied lives of those who walk the city's streets. Here, in the sanctuaries of skin refinement, the one-size-fits-all approach is replaced by a couture beauty experience, meticulously crafted to fit each client's unique narrative. It's where luxury meets personalization, and every application, every technique, is a testament to the individual's own version of Manhattan glamour.

➤ **The Consultation Chronicle: Unraveling the Personal Skincare Tale**. Every Tailored Experience begins with a consultation, a deep dive into one's personal skincare story. It's an intimate conversation, where desires and concerns are shared, setting the stage for a treatment that's as unique as the individual's own skin.

➤ **The Customized Concoction: Crafting the Personal Portion**. Imagine creams, serums, and masks, all chosen and blended to cater specifically to your skin's needs. This is alchemy at its finest, where each ingredient is handpicked, ensuring that what touches your skin is as exclusive as your fingerprint.

➤ **The Technique Tailoring: A Choreography for Your Skin**. The application techniques themselves are adapted to suit you. From gentle strokes for the sensitive soul to robust massages for the resilient, every motion is in sync with your skin's rhythm, a dance choreographed just for you.

➤ **The Evolving Elegance: Beauty that Grows with You**. As you evolve, so does your Experience. These treatments are designed to adapt to your changing skin, ensuring that your skincare journey is a continuous celebration of your individuality and elegance.

- ➢ **The Sensory Symphony: Engaging All Senses.** Each Tailored Experience is designed to engage all senses, from the soothing sounds of a curated playlist to the aromatic scents that fill the room, enhancing the overall ambiance and immersing you in a fully rejuvenating sensory experience.

- ➢ **The Follow-Up Flourish: Continued Care and Guidance.** After your session, the experience doesn't just end. You receive personalized advice and follow-up care recommendations, ensuring that the benefits of your custom treatment extend far beyond the sanctuary's doors.

- ➢ **The VIP Vault: Exclusive Access to Rare Ingredients.** Gain exclusive access to some of the most rare and potent ingredients in the world. These high-caliber elements are reserved for those who seek nothing but the best in their quest for skincare perfection.

- ➢ **The Community Connection: Part of an Elite Circle.** By participating in the Tailored Experience, you become part of an elite community of beauty aficionados who value excellence and exclusivity. This community often receives first access to new services, products, and special events.

In Manhattan's world of Tailored Experiences, skincare becomes a personal affair, a luxurious journey that honors the individuality of each patron. It's a world where every treatment is a story told, every application a verse in the poem of personal beauty. For those who step into these hallowed halls of skin refinement, the experience is more than skin deep; it's a reflection of their own unique place in the tapestry of Manhattan life. Here, in the city where uniqueness is the greatest luxury, the Tailored Experience is not just a facial; it's a celebration of the individual, a bespoke beauty ritual that's as singular and extraordinary as Manhattan itself.

# Completed Tasks: Tailored Experience Activities

_Inspirational Quote_

IT IS BY ACTS AND NOT BY IDEAS THAT PEOPLE LIVE. —— Anatole France

FIFTH AVENUE FACIALS

*Action Items: Intentions and Thoughts*

# URBAN ELIXIR

## *The Ritual of Renewal*

In the pulsating heart of Manhattan, where every moment is a whirlwind of activity, there exists a sacred ritual—the Ritual of Renewal. This is not merely a skincare routine; it's a sanctified rite, a periodic pilgrimage into the world of rejuvenation and self-care. For the denizens of this relentless city, this ritual is their secret to emerging anew, ready to embrace the city's unending tempo. Here, in the sanctuaries of serenity scattered amidst the skyscrapers, the Ritual of Renewal is an essential escape, a momentary pause where time slows, and the soul is nurtured.

➢ **The Harmonious Beginning: A Symphony of Senses**. The ritual commences with an ambiance that soothes the senses. Soft music, delicate fragrances, and a calming touch set the stage for renewal, creating an oasis of peace in the midst of Manhattan's chaos.

➢ **The Purification Process: Cleansing the Urban Canvas**. At the heart of the ritual lies the purification process. Gentle yet effective cleansing removes the traces of the city—the grime, the stress, the relentless energy—preparing the skin, and the spirit, for rejuvenation.

➢ **The Nourishing Interlude: Feeding the Skin and Soul**. Essential to the ritual is the nourishment phase, where the skin is fed with nutrients, hydration, and care. This is a moment of indulgence, where luxurious creams and serums are not just applied, but massaged deeply, ensuring every pore is a recipient of care.

➢ **The Reflective Reawakening: Emerging with Renewed Perspective**. Conclude the ritual with a moment of reawakening. This is where you slowly transition back to reality, much like the city stirs awake at dawn, refreshed and ready. It's a time to savor the renewed sense of calm and clarity, a rare treasure in the city's unceasing rhythm.

➢ **The Reflective Finale: A Moment of Quietude**. As the ritual nears its end, there's a moment of quiet reflection. It's a chance to bask in the tranquility, to absorb the serenity, to prepare for re-entry into the bustling world outside, renewed in body and spirit.

➢ **The Detoxifying Detour: Purging the Metropolitan Stress**. In this essential step, the ritual embraces detoxification techniques that purge the skin of environmental stressors. Think of clay masks and steam treatments that draw out impurities, much like the city sheds its day at twilight, preparing for the rejuvenating night.

➢ **The Energizing Elixir: A Burst of Vitality for the Skin**. Infuse the ritual with energizing elixirs—serums and essences that invigorate the skin. These concoctions are akin to the city's own energizing pulse, injecting life and vibrancy, reawakening the skin like the first light over the East River.

➢ **The Soothing Sonata: Calming the Urban Spirit**. Incorporate elements that soothe and calm. This might involve a gentle facial massage or a cooling mask, akin to a serene walk in Central Park. It's a necessary counterpoint to the city's high tempo, providing a moment of serenity amid the relentless beat of Manhattan.

In Manhattan, the Ritual of Renewal is more than a mere escape; it's a vital part of the city's rhythm, a sacred pause that allows its participants to thrive amidst the chaos. It's a testament to the belief that in order to conquer the city, one must first take a moment to rejuvenate. For those who partake in this ritual, it's not just about maintaining beauty; it's about reaffirming their connection to themselves and to the pulsating heart of the city they call home. In a place where time is the most precious commodity, the Ritual of Renewal stands as a luxurious defiance, a reminder that to truly live in the moment, one must occasionally step away from it.

## Completed Tasks: Ritual of Renewal Activities

_____
_____
_____
_____
_____
_____
_____
_____
_____
_____
_____
_____
_____
_____
_____
_____
_____
_____
_____
_____
_____
_____
_____

### Inspirational Quote

SHOW ME YOUR HANDS. DO THEY HAVE SCARS FROM GIVING? SHOW ME
YOUR FEET. ARE THEY WOUNDED IN SERVICE? SHOW ME YOUR HEART.
HAVE YOU LEFT A PLACE FOR DIVINE LOVE? — Fulton J. Sheen

*Action Items: Intentions and Thoughts*

*The Afterglow*

As the city that never sleeps slowly yields to the quiet of the night, there emerges a phenomenon known to Manhattan's beauty connoisseurs as The Afterglow. It's the radiant result of the city's coveted skincare rituals, a visible testament to the indulgent treatments and luxurious pampering that only the city's best-kept secrets can provide. This afterglow isn't merely a fleeting effect; it's a lasting impression, a glow that speaks of well-cared-for skin and a life lived in the lap of luxury. It's the mark of a Manhattanite who knows the value of self-care, embodying the vibrant energy and timeless elegance of the city in every pore.

> ➤ **The Visible Vibrance: Radiance that Speaks Volumes**. Picture stepping out into the city night, your skin not just refreshed, but visibly vibrant. This is the first hallmark of the Afterglow—a radiance that tells tales of expert care, a complexion that catches the light of every streetlamp and moonbeam.

> ➤ **The Silken Touch: Softness You Can Feel**. Then, there's the unmistakable softness, a texture as luxurious as the finest silk drapes of a Fifth Avenue penthouse. It's a tactile testament to the nourishing masks and serums, a feeling so indulgent, every touch is a reminder of the city's lavish love for skincare.

> ➤ **The Lasting Hydration: A Reservoir of Richness**. This is about hydration that endures, much like the city's relentless spirit. The skin, plumped with the finest ingredients, retains a dewy fullness that speaks of deep, lasting nourishment—a hydration that withstands the test of time and the city's elements.

> ➤ **The Refined Radiance: An Aura of Elegance**. The final facet of the Afterglow is the refined radiance, a subtle sheen that's less about shine and more about a polished, elegant aura. It's a glow that's

understated yet undeniable, a perfect blend of grace and sophistication.

➤ **The Youthful Emanation: Defying Time with Every Glimpse**. Each step into the Manhattan night reveals a youthful emanation, a skin that defies time and speaks of ageless grace. It's as if the hands of the clock have been turned back, not just through the illusion of makeup, but through the genuine restoration of the skin's youthful vigor.

➤ **The Even-Toned Elegance: A Canvas of Perfection**. Notice the even-toned elegance that the Afterglow bestows. It's like the city's skyline at sunset, flawless and awe-inspiring. This evenness isn't just about color correction; it's about achieving a naturally balanced complexion that needs no filter, just the city's ambient light

➤ **The Poreless Panache: Refinement in Every Pore**. The Afterglow brings with it a poreless panache, where each pore seems to have vanished, leaving behind a smooth canvas. It's a testament to the meticulous cleansing and refining treatments, a level of detail that mirrors the city's architectural finesse.

The Afterglow is more than a post-facial phenomenon; it's an emblem of a lifestyle, a symbol of the care and attention that Manhattanites devote to their skin. For those who walk the city's streets, this glow is a badge of honor, a sign of belonging to an exclusive world where beauty is nurtured and cherished. It's not just seen; it's envied and aspired to, a beacon of beauty that shines bright in the city of dreams. In the world of Manhattan's elite, where every detail is curated with precision, the Afterglow is the ultimate accessory, a luminous finish that complements every outfit, every occasion, every moment in the city's endless rhythm.

## Completed Tasks: Afterglow Activities

_Inspirational Quote_

HOPE IS BUT THE DREAM OF THOSE WHO WAKE. — Matthew Prior

*Action Items: Intentions and Thoughts*

*Action Items: Intentions and Thoughts*

_____
_____
_____
_____
_____
_____
_____
_____
_____
_____
_____
_____
_____
_____
_____
_____
_____
_____
_____
_____
_____
_____
_____
_____

# 7

# Tribeca Tonics:
## The Balancing Act for Lustrous, Even Tones

Ah, Manhattan—the metropolis of dreams, where shadows play on cobblestone streets, and golden sunsets bathe the skyscrapers. It's a city that demands more than mere presence; it craves a performance, a dance of daring and dexterity. In these hallowed lanes, your journey isn't just about reaching a destination; it's about the narrative you craft along the way.

Picture this: You're meandering through the heart of Tribeca, a vision of grace. Onlookers are entranced, not by the flair of your attire, but by the symphony of your skin—a harmony of hues, a testament to balance. That, my dear, is the Tribeca Tonic Touch, a signature that speaks of sophistication and the pursuit of perfection.

In this mesmerizing installment of The Manhattan Diaries, we will venture into the elusive realm of Tribeca's tonics. From elixirs steeped in age-old traditions to innovative concoctions promising equilibrium, you're about to uncover the alchemy behind the city's most sought-after skin serenades.

But understand, this is more profound than mere aesthetics. It's about turning in to Manhattan's rhythm, about presenting a face that mirrors the city's kaleidoscope—its lights, its shadows, its vibrancy, and its verve. It's about being a beacon amidst the concrete canyons and the verdant oases.

Join me as we wander through Tribeca, where every street corner whispers secrets of the past, enriching our journey and our very selves. In Manhattan, your skin doesn't just shine—it tells stories, echoing the balance and beauty of the city. Welcome to The Manhattan Diaries, where your complexion captivates as much as the city's tales. Here, beauty is more than skin deep—it's a narrative woven through every glowing face. Let's discover how each sparkle of your skin narrates the rich tapestry of Manhattan life.

*The Elixir of Evenness*

In the heart of Manhattan, where the pursuit of perfection is not just a desire but a way of life, the Elixir of Evenness reigns supreme. This isn't just any skincare concoction; it's a liquid narrative of balance and beauty, a prized potion coveted by those who walk the glamorous streets of Tribeca. The Elixir of Evenness is the answer to every city dweller's dream of flawless skin, a symbol of the relentless pursuit of an even-toned, radiant complexion that mirrors the city's own polished and poised demeanor.

➤ **The Harmonizing Ingredients: A Symphony of Skin Balance**. At the core of the Elixir of Evenness are ingredients that harmonize the skin. Think of potent botanicals and cutting-edge compounds working in tandem, reducing dark spots, and imparting a uniform glow, much like the way the city lights up at night—evenly brilliant and breathtakingly beautiful.

➤ **The Texture of Luxury: Silken Drops of Elegance**. The elixir's texture is a tale in itself. Silky, luxurious, and lightweight, it glides onto the skin like a whisper, leaving behind a feeling of opulence and comfort, as if one is draped in the finest silk gown for an evening soiree.

➤ **The Radiant Result: The Promise of Perfection**. The result of this elixir is nothing short of transformative. A complexion that speaks of evenness and luminosity, a face that tells a story of meticulous care and high-end living, a testament to the Tribeca lifestyle.

➤ **The Daily Ritual: A Moment of Manhattan Magic**. Incorporating the Elixir of Evenness into a daily skincare routine becomes a ritual, a moment to indulge in the magic of Manhattan's elite beauty secrets. It's a daily reaffirmation of one's commitment to elegance and perfection.

- ➤ **The Scent of Sophistication: A Fragrance that Tells a Story**. Each application of the Elixir of Evenness is accompanied by a subtle, enchanting fragrance. It's a scent that's not just pleasing, but evocative of the chic streets of Tribeca, reminiscent of a breezy evening walk through its sophisticated alleys.

- ➤ **The Protective Barrier: Shielding the Urban Skin**. This elixir isn't just about enhancing beauty; it's also about protection. It forms a gentle barrier against the city's environmental aggressors, much like the way the city's skyscrapers shield its inhabitants, keeping the skin as safe as it is radiant.

- ➤ **The Long-Lasting Luminosity: Glow that Goes the Distance**. The true magic of this elixir lies in its lasting power. The glow it imparts isn't fleeting but enduring, much like the timeless charm of Manhattan itself. It's a luminosity that carries one from daybreak meetings to twilight gatherings.

- ➤ **The Inclusive Radiance: A Glow for Every Skin Tone** True to Manhattan's diverse spirit, the Elixir of Evenness is designed for all skin tones. It's a celebration of the city's melting pot culture, offering a universal glow that's as inclusive as the city's vibrant populace.

The Elixir of Evenness is more than a skincare product; it's an emblem of Tribeca's skincare artistry. For the Manhattanite who uses it, it's a daily tribute to their own standards of beauty and balance, a reflection of their place in this dynamic city. Each application is not just a step in a beauty routine; it's an embrace of the luxurious, balanced lifestyle that Tribeca epitomizes. In a city where excellence is the norm, this elixir stands out as a beacon of perfection, a prized possession in the beauty arsenal of those who call Manhattan their home.

# Completed Tasks: Elixir of Evenness Activities

*Action Items: Intentions and Thoughts*

## The Tradition Meets Innovation

In the ever-evolving landscape of Manhattan, where the skyscrapers reach for the stars and the streets hum with ceaseless innovation, there lies a unique blend of beauty tradition and avant-garde science—a fusion where Tradition Meets Innovation. This is the realm where ancient skincare secrets are reimagined through the lens of modern technology, creating a symphony of treatments that are as time-honored as they are cutting-edge. It's a dance of contrasts, where the wisdom of the past gracefully waltzes with the advancements of the present, all within the luxurious confines of Tribeca's elite skincare boutiques.

> ➤ **The Herbal Revolution: Ancient Botanicals, Modern Efficacy**. Imagine herbs and plants used for centuries, now supercharged with contemporary science to maximize their skin-enhancing properties. This point explores how traditional botanicals are given new life; their natural powers amplified for today's skincare needs.

> ➤ **The Thermal Renaissance: From Hot Springs to High Tech**. Delve into the rejuvenating power of thermal therapies, once a gift of nature's hot springs, now recreated with state-of-the-art temperature control. It's a nod to the healing practices of old, revitalized with the precision and comfort of modern technology.

> ➤ **The Crystal Comeback: Timeless Stones, Trendsetting Tools**. Rediscover the mystical allure of crystals in skincare, an ancient practice now trending in the form of modern facial tools. These gemstones, steeped in historical significance, are reinterpreted to align with the contemporary quest for holistic beauty.

> ➤ **The Technological Touch: Digital Age Meets Dermatological Art**. Witness the integration of digital advancements into skincare techniques. High-tech diagnostics and treatments offer a

personalized skincare journey, blending the artisanal touch of the past with the digital precision of the present.

➤ **The Aromatic Alchemy: Scented Stories, Modern Methods**. Envelop yourself in the aromatic alchemy where age-old scents blend with modern fragrance techniques. These olfactory experiences, once a cornerstone of ancient rituals, are now enhanced to evoke emotions and memories, tailored to the urban sophisticate's desires.

➤ **The Regenerative Rituals: Historic Remedies, Today's Triumphs**. Delve into regenerative rituals that have stood the test of time, now boosted by contemporary scientific discoveries. These treatments, rooted in history, are redefined to offer enhanced skin rejuvenation, merging the best of past and present for transformative results.

➤ **Biodynamic Skincare: Ancient Cycles and Modern Science**. Explore biodynamic skincare, which merges ancient agricultural practices with contemporary biotech to create potent, earth-friendly products. This method not only utilizes natural cycles but also incorporates advanced science for effective, sustainable skincare solutions.

In the heart of Tribeca, the meeting of Tradition and Innovation in skincare forms a harmonious symphony that resonates with the rhythm of Manhattan. It's a celebration of how far we've come in the art of beauty, a testament to the city's ability to honor its past while boldly embracing the future. For the discerning Manhattanite, this fusion is not just a trend; it's a lifestyle, a seamless blend of the city's rich heritage with its dynamic progress. Here, in the city that always looks forward, beauty is a dance of timeless practices and innovative breakthroughs, creating a skincare experience that's as richly layered as Manhattan's own history.

## Completed Tasks: Tradition & Innovation Activities

_____
_____
_____
_____
_____
_____
_____
_____
_____
_____
_____
_____
_____
_____
_____
_____
_____
_____
_____
_____
_____
_____
_____
_____
_____

### Inspirational Quote

YOUR BIG OPPORTUNITY MAY BE RIGHT WHERE YOU ARE NOW. —
Napoleon Hill

# Action Items: Intentions and Thoughts

## *The Ritual of Application*

In the heart of Manhattan, where every moment pulses with a rhythm all its own, the Ritual of Application in skincare becomes a dance of elegance and precision. This isn't just the daily dabbing of creams and serums; it's a choreographed performance, a moment where the hurried pace of the city yields to the deliberate, graceful art of self-care. Here, each stroke and each pat is an expression, a testament to the belief that beauty is as much in the application as it is in the product. It's a ritual that embodies the sophistication and finesse of Manhattan, a daily indulgence that's as integral to the city's routine as the morning coffee from a favorite cafe.

➢ **The Preparatory Pause: Setting the Stage**. Before a single product touches the skin, there's a moment of preparation. It's a pause to breathe, to clear the mind, akin to the quiet hush that falls over a theater before the curtain rises. This preparatory step is essential, setting the stage for a mindful application.

➢ **The Strategic Sequence: An Order of Elegance**. Each product is applied in a strategic sequence, a thoughtful order that maximizes their efficacy. It's like the city's own symphony each element in perfect harmony, from the lightest serum to the richest cream, building towards a crescendo of skincare perfection.

➢ **The Gentle Embrace: Touch of Grace**. The manner of application is a gentle, deliberate embrace. Fingers glide and tap over skin, not just applying but massaging, ensuring each product is not just applied but absorbed, much like the way Manhattan absorbs every dream and aspiration within its borders.

➢ **The Reflective Finale: A Moment to Admire**. Concluding the ritual is a moment of reflection, a final look in the mirror to admire the work of art that is your skin. It's a celebration of the time and effort invested, a nod to the beauty and resilience reflected back.

- ➤ **The Precision of Patting: Gentle Yet Effective**. Embrace the art of patting products into the skin. This technique, refined over generations, ensures maximum absorption and effectiveness. It's a delicate yet deliberate motion, reminiscent of the gentle tapping of rain on a Manhattan penthouse window, soothing and effective.

- ➤ **The Upward Journey: Defying Gravity with Every Stroke**. Each application follows an upward trajectory, defying gravity in a city that reaches for the skies. This upward motion is symbolic of the city's own aspirations, a small but significant act of lifting and firming the skin, as Manhattan lifts the spirits of its inhabitants.

- ➤ **The Eye Area Ballet: A Dance of Delicacy**. The application around the eyes is a ballet of its own—soft, precise, and delicate. It's a dance that respects the sensitivity of the area, with each tap and dab akin to the delicate steps of a ballerina on the stage of Lincoln Center.

- ➤ **The Mindful Finale: A Moment of Gratitude**. Conclude the ritual with a moment of mindfulness, a thank you to oneself and the products that nurture the skin. It's a closing ceremony that acknowledges the luxury of self-care in a city that is perpetually on the move, a moment of gratitude for the peace found within the ritual.

In Manhattan, the Ritual of Application is a symphony of movements, a daily practice that goes beyond routine to become a moment of luxury and self-expression. It's an affirmation of the city's ethos—that beauty is crafted, nurtured, and savored. For the Manhattanite who partakes in this ritual, it's not just skincare; it's a testament to their place in this dynamic city, a harmonious blend of discipline, art, and elegance. In a city where every second counts, this ritual is a cherished interlude, a personal tribute to the timeless art of beauty.

## Completed Tasks: Application Ritual Activities

_____
_____
_____
_____
_____
_____
_____
_____
_____
_____
_____
_____
_____
_____
_____
_____
_____
_____
_____
_____
_____
_____
_____
_____
_____

### Inspirational Quote

TEARS ARE OFTEN THE TELESCOPE BY WHICH MEN SEE FAR INTO HEAVEN.
— Henry Ward Beecher

*Action Items: Intentions and Thoughts*

*The Palette of Potions*

In the bustling streets of Manhattan, where every turn reveals a new secret and every moment is an opportunity for discovery, there exists a palette of potions that are the essence of skincare alchemy. This isn't just a collection of products; it's a curated selection of magical elixirs, each a bearer of the city's stories and secrets. The Palette of Potions is a treasure trove for the skin, offering a solution for every concern and a promise for every desire. Here, amidst the glamour and the grit of the city, these potions are more than skincare; they're liquid narratives, each drop a blend of Manhattan's luxurious essence and the cutting-edge science that defines its heartbeat.

> ➢ **The Hydrating Harmonizer: Quenching the City's Thirst**. This potion is a marvel of hydration, a formula designed to imbue the skin with moisture as deeply as Central Park's Great Lawn absorbs the morning dew. It's a drink for the skin, leaving it as refreshed as the city after a spring rain.

> ➢ **The Revitalizing Reviver: Awakening with Every Application**. Like a brisk walk through the lively streets of SoHo, this potion is an energizer, reviving tired skin and invigorating it with new life. It's a wake-up call in a bottle, turning back the effects of those long city nights.

> ➢ **The Soothing Spell: Calm in the City Chaos**. Amidst the city's clamor, this potion offers a moment of calm. It soothes and repairs, much like the tranquil respite of a quiet corner in a bustling cafe, providing relief from the relentless pace of urban life.

> ➢ **The Brightening Brew: Illuminating Like the Times Square Lights**. This potion is all about radiance, offering a brightness that rivals the city's most dazzling lights. It's a formula that brings clarity and luminosity to the skin, echoing the vibrant energy of Manhattan.

- ➢ **The Anti-Aging Alchemist: Turning Back Time on Fifth Avenue**. A potion that defies time, smoothing lines and softening signs of aging, much like the timeless elegance found in the city's grandest avenues. It's a fountain of youth, bottled up in Tribeca's chicest boutiques.

- ➢ **The Firming Formula: Sculpting the Manhattan Silhouette**. Like the chiseled architecture of the city's skyline, this potion is all about firming and sculpting. It works to redefine the contours of the skin, offering a tautness and resilience that mirrors the city's unyielding spirit.

- ➢ **The Pore-Refining Potion: As Precise as a Broadway Production**. This elixir zeroes in on pores, refining them with the precision of a well-rehearsed Broadway show. It's a performance in a bottle, tightening and minimizing pores to create a smooth, flawless canvas akin to the city's polished theater stages.

- ➢ **The Luminous Lift: Elevating Like the Empire State**. This potion provides an uplifting effect, much like the awe-inspiring ascent to the top of the Empire State Building. It lifts and illuminates the skin, infusing it with a youthful, radiant glow that's visible from the city's loftiest rooftops.

The Palette of Potions in Manhattan's skincare scene is a spectrum of wonder, each potion a testament to the city's prowess in beauty and innovation. For those who delve into this palette, it's not just about addressing skin concerns; it's about embracing a lifestyle, a commitment to the art and science of beauty that Manhattan epitomizes. Each potion is a chapter in the city's ongoing story of elegance and advancement, a liquid ode to the never-ending pursuit of perfection that pulses in the heart of The Big Apple.

## Completed Tasks: Palette of Potions Activities

_____

_____

_____

_____

_____

_____

_____

_____

_____

_____

_____

_____

_____

_____

_____

_____

_____

_____

_____

_____

_____

_____

_____

_____

_____

_____

_____

_____

_____

_____

_____

_____

_____

_____

_____

_____

_____

*Inspirational Quote*

MY MIND'S MY KINGDOM. — Francis Quarles

*Action Items: Intentions and Thoughts*

## The Afterglow of Tribeca

In the enchanting enclave of Tribeca, where old-world charm meets modern luxury, there's a coveted phenomenon known intimately to the city's beauty elite—the Afterglow of Tribeca. This isn't just the result of a well-executed skincare routine; it's a radiant declaration, a visible celebration of the neighborhood's illustrious approach to beauty and self-care. The Afterglow is the whispered secret of Manhattan's most discerning, a glowing testament to the transformative power of Tribeca's skincare rituals. It's more than just skin deep; it's a reflection of the neighborhood's soul—understated, elegant, and utterly captivating.

- ➢ **The Illuminated Complexion: Radiance Worthy of Tribeca's Art Galleries**. Just as the art in Tribeca's galleries illuminates the soul, the Afterglow brightens the complexion. It's a luminosity that speaks of expert care, a glow that seems to emanate from within, mirroring the subtle sophistication of the area's cobblestoned streets and historic lofts.

- ➢ **The Velvet Texture: As Luxurious as Tribeca's Loft Living**. The Afterglow leaves the skin with a texture as smooth and luxurious as the velvet drapes adorning Tribeca's lofty interiors. It's a softness that invites touch, a testament to the nourishing potions and elixirs that are the cornerstones of Tribeca's skincare philosophy.

- ➢ **The Refined Pores: Precision in Every Detail**. In Tribeca, where attention to detail is paramount, the Afterglow reflects this ethos with refined, almost invisible pores. It's a skin texture that's as meticulously curated as the neighborhood's chic boutiques and eateries.

- ➢ **The Lasting Hydration: A Quenching as Profound as the Hudson**. The hydration that comes with the Afterglow is deep and enduring, much like the waters of the Hudson bordering this historic neighborhood. It's a moisture that locks in, keeping the skin plump and resilient, ready to face the city's challenges.

- ➤ **The Subtle Sculpting: Contours as Defined as Tribeca's Architecture**. This Afterglow isn't just about brightness; it subtly sculpts and defines, much like the distinct architectural lines of Tribeca's buildings. It's a gentle toning effect that adds dimension and depth, enhancing natural features with grace.

- ➤ **The Even-Toned Elegance: A Palette as Harmonious as Tribeca's Streets**. The Afterglow imparts an even-toned elegance, smoothing out imperfections and creating a canvas as harmonious and balanced as Tribeca's own blend of the historic and the contemporary. It's a complexion that speaks of meticulous care and understated grace.

- ➤ **The Resilient Radiance: Glow with the Endurance of City Life**. In Tribeca, resilience is key, and the Afterglow reflects this with its long-lasting radiance. This isn't a fleeting luminescence; it's a glow that endures the hustle of city life, much like the enduring spirit of the neighborhood itself.

- ➤ **The Youthful Vibrancy: A Reflection of Tribeca's Timeless Energy**. The final touch of the Afterglow is a youthful vibrancy, a reflection of the timeless, energetic spirit that pervades Tribeca.

The Afterglow of Tribeca is more than a post-facial phenomenon; it's a tribute to the neighborhood's timeless approach to beauty. For those who wear this glow, it's a symbol of a life well-lived, of evenings spent in intimate cafes and days wandering along the waterfront. It's not just an aftereffect of skincare; it's a lifestyle, a commitment to the art of self-preservation and elegance. In Tribeca, where history blends seamlessly with modernity, the Afterglow is a beacon of beauty, a radiant emblem of the neighborhood's enduring charm and sophistication.

## Completed Tasks: Afterglow of the City Activities

_____
_____
_____
_____
_____
_____
_____
_____
_____
_____
_____
_____
_____
_____
_____
_____
_____
_____
_____
_____
_____
_____
_____
_____
_____

### Inspirational Quote

WHAT MAKES THE DESERT BEAUTIFUL IS THAT SOMEWHERE IT HIDES A WELL. — Antoine de Saint-Exupery

TRIBECA TONICS

*Action Items: Intentions and Thoughts*

## Action Items: Intentions and Thoughts

# 8

# Brooklyn Bridge Barrier Creams: Crossing Over to Ultimate Hydration

Ah, Manhattan—where every boulevard tells a story, and every glance is a whispered secret. In this city of dreams and dramas, life isn't about mere survival; it's about thriving with flair, and of course, that enviable radiance. Because here, among the dazzle of neon and the glint of ambition, it's never just about where you're headed, but how glowing you embark on the journey.

Imagine: There you are, confidently navigating the concrete trails of Fifth Avenue, each step an ode to grace. Gaze upon gaze is irresistibly pulled towards you, and it's not the haute couture they're admiring—it's the luminosity of your skin, the undeniable Brooklyn Bridge Brilliance. A radiance so arresting, it can only be rivaled by the city lights themselves.

Dive deep with me in this chapter of The Manhattan Diaries, as we explore the allure behind Brooklyn Bridge Barrier Creams. These are not mere moisturizers; they're gateways to unparalleled hydration, the lifeline connecting you to the age-old secrets of the city's most radiant. Whether you're seeking a gentle embrace of moisture or a floodgate of hydration, you'll find the map to your heart's desire right here.

But let's be clear, this journey is about more than skin deep splendor. It's about reflecting the city's essence, its pulse, its thirst for life. It's about guarding your skin from the city's tales of exhaust and excitement, while still dancing freely in its embrace.

So, step forth with me, as we cross this iconic bridge of beauty, harmonizing with the rhythm of the East River below. Remember, darling, in Manhattan, every drop of hydration is a step closer to your spotlight moment. The stage is set, and the city, with bated breath, awaits your luminous debut. Welcome to The Manhattan Diaries—where your glow competes with the stars themselves.

## The Hydration Highway

In the sprawling urban landscape of Manhattan, where the pace is relentless and the air is brimming with ambition, there's an essential journey for the skin—the Hydration Highway. This isn't just a path to quenching thirsty skin; it's a route to preserving the city's most valuable asset—your face. Here, amidst the towering skyscrapers and endless avenues, Brooklyn Bridge Barrier Creams serve as your guide, leading you through a labyrinth of environmental stressors and city smog, ensuring your skin remains as hydrated as the city is energetic.

- ➢ **The Quenching Quest: Embarking on the Journey**. Begin your journey with a cream that dives deep into the skin's layers, delivering hydration that penetrates beyond the surface. It's like the city's underground, a network of moisture working tirelessly beneath the visible.

- ➢ **The Barrier Builder: Fortifying the Urban Shield**. Along the Hydration Highway, fortify your skin's natural barrier. These creams form a protective layer, much like Manhattan's towering walls, guarding against pollution, wind, and the wear of city life.

- ➢ **The Nourishing Stop: Replenishing at Every Turn**. At every corner of this journey, there's a chance to nourish. Rich in vitamins and antioxidants, these creams feed your skin, just as the city feeds the dreams of its inhabitants.

- ➢ **The Enduring Hydration: Lasting Through the City's Marathon**. The true test of any journey on the Hydration Highway is endurance. These creams ensure hydration that lasts, much like the enduring spirit of New York itself—never fading, always glowing.

- ➢ **The Soothing Stretch: A Calm Amidst the City Rush**. In this segment of the highway, find solace in the soothing properties of the creams. It's like finding a quiet park in the midst of Manhattan's hustle—a moment of calm that reduces redness and irritation, offering a peaceful respite for stressed skin.

➢ **The Revitalizing Route: Energizing with Every Application**. This point of the journey brings a burst of energy to the skin, much like a brisk walk through Times Square. Enriched with revitalizing ingredients, these creams invigorate and awaken the skin, breathing new life into tired city-worn faces.

➢ **The Deep-Dive Detour: Plunging into the Depths of Hydration**. Here, delve deeper into hydration with ingredients that mimic the skin's natural moisturizing factors. It's a dive into the essence of true hydration, ensuring that moisture is not just surface-level, but deeply ingrained, as deep as the city's roots.

➢ **The Glowing Gateway: The Final Stretch to Radiance**. As the journey nears its end, enter the gateway to a glowing complexion. This final stretch is where the creams lock in all the benefits, sealing in moisture for a radiant finish that glows as brightly as the city at golden hour.

As you conclude your journey on the Hydration Highway, you arrive at a destination of dewy, radiant skin. It's a triumph akin to conquering the city's bustling streets, a victory of resilience and care. With Brooklyn Bridge Barrier Creams, your skin becomes a reflection of Manhattan's indomitable spirit—continuously hydrated, perpetually radiant, and forever ready to face the city's next challenge. In the story of The Manhattan Diaries, this journey isn't just about skincare; it's about embracing the city's essence, one hydrated day at a time.

URBAN ELIXIR

*Completed Tasks: Hydration Highway Activities*

---

*Inspirational Quote*

EVERY CHARITABLE ACT IS A STEPPINGSTONE TOWARD HEAVEN. — Henry
Ward Beecher

152

*Action Items: Intentions and Thoughts*

## The Texture of Dreams

In the heart of Manhattan, where every touch tells a story and every sensation is a memory, the Texture of Dreams is woven into the very fabric of skincare. Brooklyn Bridge Barrier Creams offer more than mere hydration; they provide a tactile experience akin to the most luxurious of Manhattan's delights. This texture is a whisper against the skin, a caress as soft and inviting as a stroll through Central Park on a spring morning. It's the kind of indulgence that turns a daily routine into a moment of pure bliss, a sensory journey that mirrors the city's own blend of sophistication and serenity.

➢ **The Featherlight Embrace: Gentle as the City's Morning Breeze**. The creams' texture is as light as a feather, a gentle embrace that comforts the skin without overwhelming it. It's like the softest touch, a breeze that caresses your face as you wander through the quiet streets of Tribeca at dawn.

➢ **The Silken Glide: Smooth as the Jazz Notes of Harlem**. Applying these creams is akin to silk gliding over the skin. The smooth, luxurious feel is reminiscent of the smooth jazz that flows through the night air in Harlem, enveloping you in a sensation that's both soothing and exhilarating.

➢ **The Velvety Caress: Rich as the Velvet Curtains of Broadway**. Each application feels like the plush velvet curtains of a Broadway theater—rich, sumptuous, and undeniably luxurious. It's a texture that pampers the skin, leaving it feeling as cherished as the star of the show.

➢ **The Dewy Kiss: Fresh as a Raindrop on a Rooftop Garden**. The final touch is a dewy finish, not too oily, not too dry, but just right. It's like the delicate kiss of raindrops on a rooftop garden in the West Village, leaving the skin refreshed and revitalized.

- ➤ **The Creamy Cocoon: Embracing Like Central Park's Greenery**. Each application envelops the skin in a creamy cocoon, akin to the embracing greenery of Central Park. This rich, yet non-greasy texture, offers a protective embrace, shielding the skin from the urban elements while nourishing it deeply.

- ➤ **The Melt-Into-You Marvel: Fusing with the Skin's Own Texture**. The creams possess a remarkable ability to melt into the skin, merging seamlessly with its natural texture. It's akin to the city lights blending into the night sky, a perfect union that enhances without altering.

- ➤ **The Satin Sheen: Elegant as a Night at the Met**. Post-application, the skin is left with a satin sheen, a subtle glow that speaks of elegance and refinement. It's reminiscent of an evening at the Met, sophisticated and cultured, imparting a discreet yet undeniable allure.

- ➤ **The Balmy Bliss: Soothing as a Jazz Melody**. The texture of these creams offers a balmy bliss, soothing and calming the skin. This sensation is as comforting as the mellow melodies of a jazz club in Greenwich Village, providing a serene end to a bustling New York day.

In the world of Manhattan's skincare, the Texture of Dreams offered by Brooklyn Bridge Barrier Creams is more than a feature; it's a fantasy come to life. It turns the mundane act of moisturizing into a luxurious experience, a moment where the hustle of the city fades away, leaving only the soft, comforting embrace of dream-like texture. In a city where every sense is constantly awakened, these creams provide a moment of escape, a tactile journey as essential to the spirit as it is to the skin. In the narrative of The Manhattan Diaries, this texture isn't just felt; it's treasured, a beloved chapter in the city's ongoing love affair with beauty and indulgence.

## Completed Tasks: Texture of Dreams Activities

_____

_____

_____

_____

_____

_____

_____

_____

_____

_____

_____

_____

_____

_____

_____

_____

_____

_____

_____

_____

_____

_____

_____

_____

_____

_____

_____

_____

### Inspirational Quote

YOU ARE ALWAYS FREE TO CHANGE YOUR MIND AND CHOOSE A DIFFERENT FUTURE, OR A DIFFERENT PAST. — Richard Bach

*Action Items: Intentions and Thoughts*

## *The Protective Promise*

In the bustling heart of Manhattan, where the pace is relentless and the air is charged with ambition, the skin needs more than just nourishment—it needs protection. Enter the Protective Promise of Brooklyn Bridge Barrier Creams, a skincare savior that stands as a vigilant guard against the city's harsh elements. This isn't just a cream; it's an urban armor, a shield against the environmental onslaught that accompanies life in the concrete jungle. It's a promise to keep the skin as resilient and undaunted as the spirit of New York itself, allowing the city's denizens to face each day with confidence, knowing their skin is safeguarded.

➤ **The Pollution Guard: A Shield Against Urban Assault**. These creams form a barrier against pollution, much like the way Manhattan's skyscrapers stand tall against the city's hustle and bustle. They protect against the microscopic assailants of urban living, keeping the skin pure and untainted.

➤ **The Hydration Lock: Sealing in the City's Moisture**. In a city where every drop of moisture is precious, these creams lock in hydration. It's like the retaining walls of the Hudson River, holding in the essential hydration, ensuring the skin remains plump and resilient amidst the urban dryness.

➤ **The Anti-Aging Ally: Defending Against Time**. The creams also promise anti-aging benefits, defending the skin against the premature signs of aging. They are the timekeepers of the skin, much like the iconic clocks of Grand Central, keeping the skin youthful and timeless.

➤ **The Environmental Shield: Braving the Elements**. Whether it's the biting cold of winter or the sweltering heat of summer, these creams provide a protective layer against the extreme elements, akin to the city's own adaptability to the changing seasons.

- ➢ **The Soothing Sentinel: Calming the City's Frenzy**. Amidst the constant buzz of the city, these creams offer a soothing respite. They calm irritation and reduce redness, much like a tranquil walk in the quiet corners of the High Line, providing a peaceful escape from the urban frenzy.

- ➢ **The UV Vanguard: Guardian Against the Glare**. In a city where the sun reflects off skyscrapers and streets, the creams serve as a vanguard against harmful UV rays. It's like donning sunglasses before facing the bright Manhattan daylight, shielding the skin from potential damage.

- ➢ **The Anti-Stress Armor: Combatting the City's Pace**. The fast-paced Manhattan life can take a toll on the skin. These creams offer an anti-stress armor, combating the effects of a hectic lifestyle, just as a serene moment in Bryant Park can dissolve the day's tensions.

- ➢ **The Blue Light Barrier: A Shield in the Digital Age**. In an era where screens are as much a part of the city as its buildings, these creams protect against blue light exposure. It's a defense against the unseen elements of modern urban life, keeping the skin safe in the digital landscape of New York.

The Protective Promise of Brooklyn Bridge Barrier Creams is more than a feature; it's a commitment to preserving the skin's health and beauty in the face of urban challenges. In the narrative of The Manhattan Diaries, these creams are the unsung heroes, the silent sentinels that stand guard over the skin's well-being. They allow the city's residents to navigate the urban landscape with assurance, knowing their skin is as protected and fortified as Manhattan itself—ever enduring, ever radiant.

# URBAN ELIXIR

## *Completed Tasks: Protective Promise Activities*

---

*Inspirational Quote*

IF LIFE HAD A SECOND EDITION, HOW I WOULD CORRECT THE PROOFS. ——
John Clare

*Action Items: Intentions and Thoughts*

## The Luminous Legacy

In the illustrious cityscape of Manhattan, where every corner is steeped in history and every face tells a story, the pursuit of a radiant complexion is more than a desire—it's a legacy. The Luminous Legacy, brought to life by Brooklyn Bridge Barrier Creams, is a testament to this enduring quest for radiance. It's not just about achieving a fleeting brightness; it's about cultivating a glow that is as integral to one's identity as their signature style. This luminosity is a reflection of the city itself—vibrant, resilient, and unforgettably brilliant.

> ➤ **The Radiance Revealer: Unveiling the Inner Light**. Just as the city lights illuminate Manhattan's nights, these creams reveal the skin's inner radiance. They work to uncover a natural glow, enhancing the skin's inherent beauty, much like how the city's energy brings out the best in its inhabitants.

> ➤ **The Even-Tone Enhancer: Harmonizing the Complexion's Palette**. The creams are artisans of evenness, harmonizing the complexion much like a well-conducted symphony. They diminish the appearance of dark spots and redness, creating a canvas as balanced and graceful as the city's architectural harmony.

> ➤ **The Dewy Demeanor: A Touch of Morning Mist**. This legacy imparts a dewy finish to the skin, reminiscent of Manhattan in the gentle morning mist. It's a look that's fresh, youthful, and alive—a dewy demeanor that speaks of vitality and a city that's always in motion.

> ➤ **The Age-Defying Aura: Defying Time with Elegance**. Just as Manhattan's timeless charm weaves through its modern streets, these creams imbue the skin with an age-defying aura. They help to smooth fine lines and wrinkles, ensuring the skin remains as enduringly elegant as the city's everlasting allure.

➤ **The Hydration Highlight: Quenching the City's Thirst for Glow**. These creams not only hydrate but also illuminate. Each application is like a refreshing drink for the skin, leaving it not just moisturized but luminously hydrated, echoing the vibrant life force that pulses through the city's veins.

➤ **The Texture Transformer: Refining for a Radiant Sheen**. The transformative texture of the creams plays a pivotal role. Silky and enriching, they refine the skin's surface, leaving a radiant sheen that mirrors the polished facade of Manhattan's grandest buildings, an architectural glow brought to life on your skin.

➤ **The Antioxidant Alchemy: Fighting the Urban Fading**. Infused with antioxidants, these creams combat the dulling effects of urban living. It's a protective alchemy that preserves the skin's brightness against the backdrop of the city's challenges, much like the enduring art found in Manhattan's museums.

➤ **The Signature Scent: A Fragrance as Memorable as the City**. The final touch in this luminous legacy is the creams' signature scent. It's a fragrance that lingers, as memorable and captivating as the city itself, leaving an impression that's as lasting as the glow it imparts.

The Luminous Legacy of Brooklyn Bridge Barrier Creams is more than a skincare achievement; it's an embodiment of Manhattan's spirit. This radiance is a tribute to the city that never sleeps, a reflection of its undying energy and elegance. For those who walk the streets of Manhattan, this legacy is not just worn; it's lived. It's a luminous testament to the city's perennial charm, a glow that resonates with the timeless allure of New York—a city where beauty, like its skyline, is always reaching new heights.

# URBAN ELIXIR

*Completed Tasks: Luminously Hydrated Activities*

---

*Inspirational Quote*

TO ME, IF LIFE BOILS DOWN TO ONE THING, IT'S MOVEMENT. TO LIVE IS
TO KEEP MOVING. — Jerry Seinfeld

*Action Items: Intentions and Thoughts*

*Action Items: Intentions and Thoughts*

# 9

# Upper East Side Elixirs: Nightly Rituals for Maximum Regeneration

Manhattan—a glittering realm of enigmas, where every window pane holds a secret, and each midnight moonbeam tells tales of whispered dreams. Amidst the unending fervor of this city, it's not merely about surviving another New York minute; it's about reviving and renewing in those stolen, sultry moments after dusk—with an elegance only the Upper East Side can master.

Picture this: The sun has taken its final bow over the Hudson, and as you elegantly tread down Fifth Avenue, the world seems to stand still. They're not ensnared by the designer ensemble you don; instead, they're captivated by the rejuvenated glow of your skin—the Upper East Side Elixir Effect, if you will. It's the hush-hush ritual that makes even the most fatigued Manhattanite look as if they've stolen hours from the night.

In this beguiling chapter of The Manhattan Diaries, we unravel the mystique of the Upper East Side's nightly regimens. From potent potions that revitalize and restore to sultry serums that promise dreams distilled into every drop, here you'll unlock the quintessence of nocturnal renewal.

But this tale isn't just about beauty elixirs. Oh no, darling. It's about syncing with the city's moonlit tempo; it's about romancing the night and making love to the dawn. It's about the promise that even after the most grueling of days, the night holds the power to heal, to transform, to regenerate.

So, saunter with me under the canopy of Manhattan's starlit skies, as we indulge in rituals that don't just promise a new dawn but a reborn you. Because in this city, every evening offers a fresh start, a new script. The night is young, and the city, with its shimmering skyline, yearns for your renewed brilliance. Welcome to The Manhattan Diaries—where by daybreak, you're not just reborn, but redefined.

## *The Midnight Restoration*

In the heart of Manhattan, where the city's relentless energy meets the allure of the night, lies a secret world—the Midnight Restoration. Picture this: The clock strikes midnight, and as you traverse the bustling streets, a realm of secrets and rejuvenation unveils itself. Join me in this enchanting chapter of The Manhattan Diaries as we dive into the art of nighttime renewal, exploring the elixirs and rituals that promise to awaken your spirit. But it's not just about skincare; it's a celebration of the night, a promise of new beginnings, and the enchantment that envelops the city after dark. Welcome to The Manhattan Diaries, where the midnight hour becomes a rendezvous with transformation and rebirth.

- **The Midnight Serums**. When the moon takes center stage, the Midnight Serums step in, like secret agents of rejuvenation. These potent elixirs promise to undo the day's stress, leaving your skin refreshed and ready for a new adventure. Imagine the allure of waking up with the radiant glow of a night well-spent.

- **Sultry Nighttime Rituals**. The Upper East Side knows how to set the stage for nightly transformation. Dive into sultry nighttime rituals that make you feel like a star preparing for a red-carpet event. These are moments of self-indulgence, where skincare becomes an intimate affair with the city itself.

- **Moonlit Dream Elixirs**. The city's dreamers have distilled their aspirations into Moonlit Dream Elixirs, and they're ready to share them with you. These luxurious concoctions are designed to immerse your skin in dreams, nourishing it with the promise of a fresh start. Picture yourself as a canvas, awaiting the artistry of the night.

- **The Night's Secret Promise**. The night in Manhattan is a secret promise, a chance to hit the reset button and emerge anew. As we delve into the realm of Midnight Restoration, remember that each night is a story waiting to be written, and with the right elixirs and rituals, you're the author of your own transformation. When the dawn breaks, you'll step into the city's embrace with renewed confidence and luminosity, ready for the next chapter in The Manhattan Diaries.

➤ **Starlit Skincare Soirees**. Experience the Upper East Side's penchant for glamour with starlit skincare soirees. These gatherings are where Manhattan's elite come together to exchange their most coveted beauty secrets. Join the nocturnal beauty society and indulge in rituals that elevate your skincare routine to an art form.

➤ **A Love Letter to Yourself**. The Midnight Restoration is your nightly love letter to yourself. It's a reminder that self-care isn't just a routine; it's an act of self-love. By embracing these rituals, you're not only enhancing your skin but also nourishing your soul, ensuring that you wake up each morning feeling like a Manhattan masterpiece.

In the heart of Manhattan, where the city's relentless energy meets the allure of the night, lies a secret world—the Midnight Restoration. Picture this: The clock strikes midnight, and as you traverse the bustling streets, a realm of secrets and rejuvenation unveils itself. Join me in this enchanting chapter of The Manhattan Diaries as we dive into the art of nighttime renewal, exploring the elixirs and rituals that promise to awaken your spirit. But it's not just about skincare; it's a celebration of the night, a promise of new beginnings, and the enchantment that envelops the city after dark. Welcome to The Manhattan Diaries, where the midnight hour becomes a rendezvous with transformation and rebirth. As dawn breaks, remember that each night holds the potential for a fresh start, allowing you to emerge renewed and redefined in the ever-evolving city that never sleeps.

## *Completed Tasks: Midnight Restoration Activities*

---
---
---
---
---
---
---
---
---
---
---
---
---
---
---
---
---
---
---
---
---
---
---
---
---
---
---
---
---
---

*Inspirational Quote*

OUR ENTIRE LIFE—CONSISTS ULTIMATELY IN ACCEPTING OURSELVES AS WE ARE. — Jean Anouilh

*Action Items: Intentions and Thoughts*

## The Dream Infusions

In the ceaseless energy of Manhattan, dreams fuel ambition and spark transformation. Envision walking through Central Park, the city's pulse softly echoing around you, as you harness the power of Dream Infusions—your secret to turning desires into reality. In this captivating section of The Manhattan Diaries, discover the alchemy of dream manifestation through visualization and intention. This journey is more than achieving goals; it's about living the dream that makes Manhattan mesmerizing.

> ➤ **The Art of Visualization**. In Manhattan, dreams take shape amidst the skyscrapers. Learn the art of visualization, a powerful technique to manifest your desires. Just as architects visualize buildings before constructing them, you can visualize your dreams coming to life against the backdrop of the city's skyline.

> ➤ **The Magic of Intention**. Intentions are like the compass guiding your dreams in Manhattan's labyrinthine streets. Discover how setting clear intentions can steer your life's course towards success and fulfillment. Let the city's energy amplify your intentions, making them even more potent.

> ➤ **Networking in Dreamland**. Manhattan is a city of connections, and the same applies to your dreams. Explore the art of networking in dreamland, where your aspirations can intersect with the dreams of others. Collaborate, exchange ideas, and watch your dreams grow exponentially.

> ➤ **The City's Inspiration**. Manhattan is an endless source of inspiration. Whether you're strolling through its iconic neighborhoods, visiting museums, or simply people-watching, the city offers a wealth of inspiration for your dreams. Let the city's vibrancy and diversity infuse your aspirations with new perspectives.

➤ **Living the Dream**. Ultimately, the Dream Infusions are about living your dreams in the heart of Manhattan. Embrace the belief that your dreams are not distant fantasies but tangible realities waiting to be realized. The city itself is proof that dreams can come true, and it's time for your dreams to shine amid the city lights.

➤ **Nocturnal Nurturing.** Embrace the transformative power of night in Manhattan, where the city's lesser-known nighttime routines foster rejuvenation. Learn how the city's most influential figures harness the quiet hours for personal growth and reflection, turning the stillness of night into a productive sanctuary.

➤ **Secrets of the Moonlit Metropolis.** Discover the hidden gems and secret spots in Manhattan that come alive at midnight, offering unique experiences and opportunities for inspiration that are unseen during the daylight hours. From exclusive night galleries to underground music sessions, these are the places where the city's magic is most potent.

➤ **The Rituals of Renewal.** Explore the specialized rituals that Manhattanites perform at night to reset and prepare for the challenges of the next day. From sophisticated skincare regimens to meditative practices by the river, these rituals are designed to align with the city's pulsating energy and enhance personal well-being.

In the whirlwind that is Manhattan, the dreams you nurture echo the city's vibrant pulse. The Manhattan Diaries invites you to transform your aspirations into reality, leveraging the city's dynamic energy. Embrace Manhattan not just as a backdrop but as a catalyst that molds your deepest desires into tangible achievements. Here, dreams are not merely dreamt; they are actively lived and realized. Welcome to a place where your ambitions are as limitless as the city's skyline.

*Completed Tasks: Dream Infusion Activities*

---

---

---

---

---

---

---

---

---

---

---

---

---

---

---

---

---

---

---

---

---

---

---

---

---

---

---

---

*Inspirational Quote*

LIFE IS A LONG LESSON IN HUMILITY. — James M. Barrier

*Action Items: Intentions and Thoughts*

## The Silken Touch

In the heart of Manhattan, where the city's pulse beats strongest, there's a secret that the elite have mastered—the art of the Silken Touch. Imagine strolling down Fifth Avenue, where every glance, every step, and every interaction is an opportunity to leave your mark. It's not just about the luxurious fabrics that adorn you; it's about the confidence, grace, and allure that exude from your every move. The Silken Touch is the embodiment of Manhattan's sophistication, a symbol of understated elegance that sets you apart in this city of dreams. Join me on this journey through The Manhattan Diaries as we delve into the world of couture, craftsmanship, and cultivating a presence that's as captivating as the city itself.

➢ **The Language of Luxury**. Just as Manhattanites speak a language of ambition, learn the nuances of luxury. Understand the craftsmanship, quality, and details that elevate your style.

➢ **The Confidence Couture**. Confidence is your best accessory. Discover how to wear it with pride, whether you're stepping into a corporate boardroom or attending a glamorous soiree.

➢ **Curating Your Signature Style**. In a city where individuality thrives, find your signature style that reflects your personality and aspirations. Create a wardrobe that tells your story.

➢ **The Art of Accessorizing**. Accessories are the punctuation marks of fashion. Learn how to choose the perfect pieces that enhance your look and make a statement.

➢ **The Power of Tailoring**. Tailoring is the secret weapon of the style-savvy in Manhattan. Dive into the world of bespoke tailoring and discover how custom-fitted clothing can take your look to the next level. From perfectly tailored suits to dresses that accentuate your curves, understanding the art of tailoring ensures that every piece in your wardrobe fits you like a glove.

➢ **Fashion Forward: Trends vs. Timeless**. Manhattan is a city where fashion trends are born and celebrated. Learn how to navigate the ever-changing world of fashion while maintaining a timeless and classic style. Explore the concept of investment pieces that stand the test of time and how to incorporate them into your wardrobe.

➢ **Wardrobe Essentials for Every Season**. Manhattan experiences a range of seasons, each requiring a different approach to style. Discover the essential pieces you need for every season, from chic winter coats to breezy summer dresses. Stay prepared for any weather while looking effortlessly stylish.

➢ **The Social Scene: Dressing for Events**. Manhattan's social calendar is packed with events, from gala fundraisers to intimate soirees. Explore the art of dressing appropriately for various occasions and venues. Whether you're attending a high-profile charity ball or a rooftop cocktail party, know how to make an entrance that leaves a lasting impression.

In Manhattan, where first impressions are everything and style is a form of self-expression, the Silken Touch isn't just a fashion statement; it's a way of life. Embrace the allure of sophistication, master the language of luxury, and curate a style that speaks volumes about who you are and where you're headed. As you embark on this transformative journey, watch in delight as the city responds to your newfound presence and allure. Welcome to The Manhattan Diaries, where your journey to sophistication and self-discovery begins.

## Completed Tasks: Silken Touch Activities

_____

_____

_____

_____

_____

_____

_____

_____

_____

_____

_____

_____

_____

_____

_____

_____

_____

_____

_____

_____

_____

_____

_____

_____

_____

_____

_____

### Inspirational Quote

LIFE IS PLEASANT. DEATH IS PEACEFUL. IT'S THE TRANSITION THAT'S TROUBLESOME. — Isaac Asimov

*Action Items: Intentions and Thoughts*

## The Radiant Awakening

Manhattan, a city that awakens with a shimmering promise every morning, where every sunrise hints at the potential for a radiant day. In this metropolis of dreams, beauty isn't just a standard; it's a way of life—a daily ritual of transformation and self-expression. As the sun kisses the skyline, we delve into the Radiant Awakening, a journey through the art of morning beauty and the secrets of day-to-night transformations. From skincare routines that elevate your glow to makeup looks that define your presence, Manhattan's radiant awakening is an ode to embracing your inner and outer beauty.

- ➢ **The Beauty of Morning Rituals**. In the heart of Manhattan, mornings are a precious canvas for self-care and rejuvenation. Dive into the world of morning beauty rituals that set the tone for your day. From indulgent skincare routines that leave your skin glowing to the subtle power of a well-chosen fragrance that lingers in the air, discover how to start your day feeling confident and looking radiant. In a city where first impressions matter, your morning beauty regimen becomes a daily act of self-love.

- ➢ **Effortless Daytime Glamour**. Manhattan's vibrant daytime pulse demands an effortless yet glamorous appearance. Explore the secrets of daytime beauty, where looking polished is an art form. From selecting makeup looks that are office-appropriate to choosing outfits that seamlessly transition from business meetings to lunch dates, learn how to navigate the city's challenges while maintaining a sophisticated and polished appearance. In Manhattan, the daytime is your runway, and elegance is your signature.

- ➢ **The Magic of Evening Transformations**. As the sun sets over the city, Manhattan transforms into a playground of glamour and sophistication. Delve into the art of evening beauty, where your look can evolve from busy-day chic to captivating night allure. Discover the secrets of sultry makeup that accentuates your features and elegant hairstyles that complement your evening attire. In the city that never sleeps, your evening transformation is a testament to your style and grace.

➤ **Nighttime Skincare Rituals**. Behind the glittering facade of Manhattan's nightlife lies the importance of nighttime skincare rituals. Explore the world of luxurious skincare products that work their magic while you sleep, ensuring you wake up with a youthful and radiant complexion. In a city that thrives on constant activity, your nighttime skincare routine becomes a vital part of preserving your beauty.

➤ **Embracing the Power of Skincare**. Manhattan's beauty aficionados understand that a flawless makeup look begins with impeccable skincare. Explore the world of serums, moisturizers, and treatments that are tailored to your skin's needs. From addressing city-induced stress to achieving that coveted Manhattan glow, discover the transformative power of skincare that paves the way for radiant beauty.

➤ **Effortless Hairstyles for the Manhattanite**. In a city known for its fast pace, your hairstyle should effortlessly keep up with your lifestyle. Dive into the realm of versatile and chic hairstyles that are suitable for the modern Manhattanite.

In Manhattan, where every moment is an opportunity to shine, your beauty rituals are your secret weapons. The Radiant Awakening is an ode to embracing the art of awakening, transforming, and radiating your inner and outer beauty. From the golden mornings to the enchanting nights, Manhattan awaits your radiant presence, ready to reflect the beauty that lies within and around you. Embrace the city's radiant awakening, for here, your beauty is as timeless as the skyline itself.

# Completed Tasks: Radiant Awakening Activities

_____
_____
_____
_____
_____
_____
_____
_____
_____
_____
_____
_____
_____
_____
_____
_____
_____
_____
_____
_____
_____
_____
_____
_____
_____
_____
_____
_____
_____

## Inspirational Quote

THE GREATEST TRAP IN OUR LIFE IS NOT SUCCESS, POPULARITY, OR POWER, BUT SELF-REJECTION. — Henri Nouwen

*Action Items: Intentions and Thoughts*

*Action Items: Intentions and Thoughts*

# 10

# NYC Nightcap:
## Embracing Sleep, the Skin's Best Kept Secret

Manhattan—a city that never truly sleeps, where the allure of twinkling skyscrapers beckons even the most weary-eyed to engage in just one more nocturnal escapade. Amidst this never-ending buzz, it's not simply about navigating the labyrinth of streets and stories; it's about how you awaken the next day—with a glow that outshines the morning sun and an energy rivaling the city's electric pulse.

Envision this: As you make your way down Fifth Avenue, dawn still an hour away, the world doesn't just see you—it feels you. Not because of the decadence of your evening attire, but the rested radiance that emanates from your very pores. That darling, is the Manhattan Midnight Magic, a testament that even in this city that never sleeps, true beauty lies in the embrace of a restful night.

In this intoxicating chapter of The Manhattan Diaries, we dive deep into the city's nighttime rituals. From the silk of a sleep mask to the allure of a lavender-scented room, you'll learn the tantalizing secrets behind achieving that post-slumber glow, even amidst the city's cacophony.

But don't be mistaken, it's not merely about shutting one's eyes to the world. It's about harmonizing with Manhattan's silent sonatas, the ones that play in the still of the night. It's about sinking into dreams while surrounded by the symphony of sirens, understanding the poetic balance between the city's relentless drive and its serene moments of reprieve.

Come with me, and we'll wander through the hushed avenues of the night, seeking the serenades that lull the city to rest, ensuring you not only walk with allure by day but rejuvenate with purpose by night. For in Manhattan, every close of the eyes is a prelude to tomorrow's magnificent performance. Welcome to The Manhattan Diaries—where your dawn radiance is as spellbinding as the city's shimmering horizon.

## The Art of Beauty Sleep

In the bustling streets of Manhattan, where the city's heartbeat never truly fades, there exists a hidden art form, cherished by the city's elite. It's the Art of Beauty Sleep, a nightly ritual that transforms ordinary slumber into a rejuvenating masterpiece.

➤ **The Silk Embrace**. Begin your journey to beauty sleep by embracing the luxurious touch of silk. Slip into the finest silk sleepwear, letting its soft caress cradle you as you drift into the world of dreams. The gentle, silky embrace not only pampers your skin but also enhances your comfort, ensuring a night of uninterrupted rest.

➤ **A Symphony of Scents**. Transform your bedroom into a haven of tranquility with scents that soothe the soul. Lavender, chamomile, and other calming fragrances can lull you into a peaceful slumber, amidst the city's nocturnal symphony. These aromatic notes create a serene ambiance, setting the stage for a night of blissful sleep.

➤ **The Pillow Palace**. Choose your pillows wisely, for they are your companions in the realm of dreams. Opt for ones that cradle your head and neck, ensuring a comfortable and restful night's sleep. The right pillows provide the necessary support, helping you awaken without the stiffness that often accompanies a night's rest.

➤ **Nocturnal Nourishment**. Incorporate a nighttime skincare ritual that nourishes your skin while you sleep. High-quality serums and creams can work their magic, leaving you with a radiant morning complexion. This beauty regimen allows you to wake up with skin that feels refreshed and revitalized, even in the heart of Manhattan's relentless pace.

➤ **Silken Dreams**. Slip beneath the silken sheets that adorn your bed, letting the luxurious fabric kiss your skin. Silk not only feels divine but also reduces friction on your hair and skin, minimizing the chances of waking up with creases and bedhead. It's a secret weapon to maintain your morning allure.

➤ **Moonlit Meditation**. Before sleep, indulge in a brief session of moonlit meditation. Find a quiet spot by your window, bathed in the silvery glow of the city's night lights. Take a few moments to center yourself, release the day's stress, and welcome the serenity of the night. This meditative pause allows you to drift into sleep with a tranquil mind.

➤ **The Sound of Slumber**. Create a soundscape that lulls you into deep slumber. Invest in a white noise machine or play gentle, soothing music that drowns out the city's nocturnal symphony. This auditory cocoon ensures that you remain undisturbed, wrapped in the soothing embrace of sleep.

➤ **The Sweet Surrender**. Lastly, surrender to the night, allowing Manhattan's energy to serenade you to sleep. In the city that never sleeps, the art of beauty sleep is your secret weapon, ensuring you wake up each day with the allure and grace of a Manhattan star. Embrace the night, my dear, for in its embrace lies the enchanting chapter of beauty sleep, ready to script your next captivating scene in The Manhattan Diaries.

So, my dear, come, let's explore the Art of Beauty Sleep and discover how to wake up each day in Manhattan with a glow that rivals the city's brightest lights. In this world of dreams and desires, beauty sleep is the enchanting chapter that ensures you're always ready for the next captivating scene in The Manhattan Diaries.

# URBAN ELIXIR

*Completed Tasks: Beauty Sleep Activities*

---
_____
_____
_____
_____
_____
_____
_____
_____
_____
_____
_____
_____
_____
_____
_____
_____
_____
_____
_____
_____
_____
_____
_____
_____
_____
_____
_____

*Inspirational Quote*

AS PEOPLE ARE WALKING ALL THE TIME, IN THE SAME SPOT, A PATH APPEARS. — John Locke

*Action Items: Intentions and Thoughts*

## Bedroom Sanctuary

In the heart of Manhattan, where the city's relentless energy pulsates through every street, your bedroom is your sanctuary—a respite from the chaos and a cocoon of comfort. It's not just a place for rest; it's your personal haven where dreams are born and secrets are whispered to the night. So, let's dive into the art of creating a bedroom sanctuary that reflects your style, rejuvenates your spirit, and rekindles your allure.

➤ **A Palette of Serenity**. Imagine your bedroom bathed in the softest hues of blue, blush, and pale gray. These colors create a serene canvas that's not just soothing to the eyes but also reminiscent of the city's skyline at dusk. It's like having your own personal piece of Manhattan right in your bedroom.

➤ **Luxurious Linens**. Picture sinking into a bed adorned with Egyptian cotton sheets so soft they feel like a caress. The high thread count ensures a silky embrace that's simply irresistible. And let's not forget the plush duvet and fluffy pillows—each night's sleep becomes a luxurious escape in the heart of the city.

➤ **Ambient Alchemy**. Imagine the gentle flicker of dimmable bedside lamps or the soft glow of candles casting enchanting shadows on your bedroom walls. The lighting sets the mood for relaxation after a bustling day in Manhattan. And the scents of lavender or jasmine? They transport you to a serene oasis, making your bedroom a true sensory sanctuary.

➤ **Cozy Corners**. Visualize a cozy reading nook with an inviting armchair and a stack of captivating books. It's a corner of your sanctuary where you can escape into other worlds. And your vanity? It's not just for getting ready; it's a space for self-care and reflection, adding depth to your bedroom's allure.

➤ **Artful Arrangement**. Think about your bedroom as your personal art gallery. Create a gallery wall with your favorite prints, or feature a statement piece that speaks to your soul. Your bedroom isn't just a place to sleep; it's a canvas where you express your style and personality.

➤ **Sensational Scents**. Envision diffusers or scented candles filling the air with fragrances that transport you to the heart of nature or the depths of a tranquil forest. Scents like eucalyptus, cedarwood, or citrus evoke a sense of calm, making your bedroom an aromatic haven where you can unwind.

➤ **Music of the Night**. Picture a Bluetooth speaker softly playing your favorite jazz tunes or soothing classical melodies. The right music can set the tone for relaxation and help you escape into a world of serenity, turning your bedroom into a private concert hall.

➤ **Textures to Touch**. Imagine a bed adorned with a variety of textured pillows, from velvety to silky to knitted. The play of textures adds depth and coziness to your sleeping space, inviting you to indulge in tactile sensations that soothe your senses.

➤ **Personalized Sanctuary**. Think about incorporating personal touches like framed photos, mementos, or artwork that hold sentimental value. These items infuse your bedroom with personality and warmth, making it a true sanctuary that reflects your journey.

Your Bedroom Sanctuary is more than just a place to lay your head; it's where you recharge, dream, and emerge each morning with the allure that's uniquely yours. In Manhattan, where the pace is relentless, your sanctuary becomes an essential part of maintaining your grace and poise. It's your haven amidst the whirlwind—a place where even in the heart of the city, you find solace and allure. Welcome to The Manhattan Diaries, where your sanctuary is your secret weapon for conquering the urban jungle with style-elegance.

# Completed Tasks: Bedroom Sanctuary Activities

_____

_____

_____

_____

_____

_____

_____

_____

_____

_____

_____

_____

_____

_____

_____

_____

_____

_____

_____

_____

_____

_____

_____

_____

## Inspirational Quote

ONLY THOSE WHO HAVE LEARNED THE POWER OF SINCERE AND SELFLESS CONTRIBUTION EXPERIENCE LIFE'S DEEPEST JOY: TRUE FULFILLMENT. — Tony Robbins

## Action Items: Intentions and Thoughts

*The Power of Mindful Rest*

Picture starting your day with a mindful awakening. Before diving into the hustle and bustle of the external world, you carve out a precious moment for yourself. As the first light of dawn filters through your window, you sit in quiet reflection. You breathe deeply, set intentions for the day ahead, and savor the simple pleasures of the morning—a warm cup of tea, the gentle chirping of birds, or the soft caress of sunlight on your skin. This morning mindfulness ritual empowers you to commence your day with clarity, purpose, and a sense of serenity that lingers long after you've left your sanctuary.

> ➢ **The Serene Sleep Sanctuary**. Imagine transforming your bedroom into a serene sleep sanctuary, where every detail is designed to promote restorative slumber. Soft, muted colors adorn the walls, creating a soothing ambiance. Plush bedding envelopes you in comfort, while minimalist decor reduces visual clutter. This harmonious environment wraps you in a cocoon of calmness, making it easier to drift into the depths of rejuvenating sleep.

> ➢ **A Nightly Unplug Ritual**. Envision a nightly ritual where you consciously disconnect from the digital world. No screens, no notifications—just you and your thoughts. As you set aside your devices, you free yourself from the constant stream of information and allow your mind to unwind. This deliberate act of unplugging becomes a sacred moment of detachment, fostering mental clarity and inner peace as you prepare to embrace the realm of dreams.

> ➢ **The Guided Meditation Voyage**. Think of a guided meditation session before bedtime as a tranquil journey to relaxation. With closed eyes, you listen to a soothing voice that leads you through a mental landscape of serenity. Your thoughts dissipate, stress melts away, and your body sinks into a state of profound calm. This

practice becomes your gateway to a night of profound and restorative sleep.

- ➢ **Dream Journaling by Moonlight**. Imagine keeping a dream journal by your bedside, ready to capture the ethereal tales woven in the tapestry of your sleep. In the soft glow of moonlight, you pick up your journal and pen, allowing the faint shimmer of lunar beams to guide your words. As you record your dreams and nighttime musings, you not only enhance your self-awareness but also create a tangible connection to the mysteries of the night.

- ➢ **The Morning Mindfulness Awakening**. Picture starting your day with mindfulness. Before rushing into the chaos of the world, you take a moment to breathe, set intentions, and savor the simple pleasures of the morning. It's a powerful way to begin your day with clarity and purpose.

- ➢ **Moonlit Reflections by the Window**. Imagine spending moments of moonlit reflection by your bedroom window. As you gaze at the silvery glow of the moon, you contemplate the mysteries of the night. It's a meditative pause that connects you to the celestial rhythms and allows you to find solace in the tranquil beauty of the nighttime world.

In the tender embrace of these additional practices, your bedroom becomes a haven of sensory delight, your sleep a luxurious experience, and your nights a canvas for celestial contemplation and self-affirmation. It's an exquisite tapestry of rituals that enrich your sleep journey, making every night a celebration of serenity and self-care. Welcome to the art of beauty sleep, where the world of dreams becomes a sanctuary for your soul, and each night is an opportunity to awaken to your inner radiance.

# URBAN ELIXIR

## Completed Tasks: Mindful Rest Activities

_____
_____
_____
_____
_____
_____
_____
_____
_____
_____
_____
_____
_____
_____
_____
_____
_____
_____
_____
_____
_____
_____
_____
_____
_____
_____
_____
_____

### Inspirational Quote

THE MAN WHO HAS NO INNER-LIFE IS A SLAVE TO HIS SURROUNDINGS. —
Henri Frederic Amiel

*Action Items: Intentions and Thoughts*

## *Late-Night Indulgences*

In the city that never sleeps, the night holds a certain allure. It's a time when the streets shimmer with the glow of neon lights, and the air is filled with whispered secrets and unspoken desires. Late-Night Indulgences are a rite of passage for those who seek to capture the essence of Manhattan after dark. In this chapter of The Manhattan Diaries, we explore the art of late-night indulgences—the moments of enchantment, the hidden gems, and the decadent delights that make the midnight hour in the city so irresistibly alluring.

- ➤ **The Midnight Meanderings**. Imagine taking a midnight meandering through the cobblestone streets of the West Village. The hush of the night amplifies the echoes of your footsteps, creating a symphony of solitude. It's a time when the city's secrets seem to come alive, and you become a part of its whispered tales. These late-night strolls are a dance with the city's mysteries, a chance to uncover its hidden gems, and a reminder that even in the darkness, there is beauty to be found.

- ➤ **Sip and Savor Under Starlight**. Picture yourself at a rooftop bar, sipping a perfectly crafted cocktail under the starlit sky. The cityscape stretches out before you, a tapestry of lights and dreams. The night air carries a sense of freedom, and every sip is a taste of possibility. It's a moment of indulgence where you savor the flavors and the view, a celebration of the city's vibrant nightlife, and a reminder that in Manhattan, the night is always young.

- ➤ **The Speakeasy Whispers**. Envision stepping into a hidden speakeasy, where the dimly lit ambiance and the smooth jazz create an atmosphere of intrigue. The bartender crafts cocktails with precision, and the conversations are laced with a hint of mystery. It's a world where secrets are shared in hushed tones, and you become a part of a timeless narrative. These late-night encounters are a journey into the city's clandestine side, a chance to be part of its underground history, and a reminder that in Manhattan, there's always more to discover.

➤ **The Midnight Muse**. Imagine finding inspiration in the quiet of the night. Whether it's writing, painting, or simply reflecting on life's mysteries, the midnight hour becomes your muse. The city's energy is palpable, and it fuels your creativity. It's a time when ideas flow freely, and you become the artist of your own narrative. These late-night moments are a source of inspiration, a reminder of the city's creative spirit, and a testament to the endless possibilities that unfold after dark.

➤ **The Midnight Melodies**. Picture yourself in a cozy jazz club tucked away in the heart of Harlem. The sultry notes of a saxophone fill the room, and the singer's voice carries stories of love and longing. It's a moment when music becomes a time machine, transporting you to the golden age of jazz. These late-night melodies are a tribute to the city's rich musical history, a chance to lose yourself in the rhythm, and a reminder that in Manhattan, the night is alive with song.

In the world of late-night indulgences, Manhattan opens its arms to those who seek adventure, flavor, art, and serenity after dark. It's a time when the city's diversity shines, its creativity thrives, and its allure deepens. Late-night indulgences are a tribute to Manhattan's multifaceted soul, a chance to explore its many facets, and a reminder that in the city that never sleeps, the night is a treasure trove of experiences waiting to be uncovered. Welcome to The Manhattan Diaries—where every late-night escapade is a chapter in the story of the city.

## Completed Tasks: Night Indulgences Activities

_____

_____

_____

_____

_____

_____

_____

_____

_____

_____

_____

_____

_____

_____

_____

_____

_____

_____

_____

_____

_____

_____

_____

_____

_____

_____

_____

_____

_____

_____

*Inspirational Quote*

THE TRUE OBJECT OF ALL HUMAN LIFE IS PLAY. EARTH IS A TASK GARDEN;
HEAVEN IS A PLAYGROUND. — Gilbert K. Chesteron

*Action Items: Intentions and Thoughts*

*Action Items: Intentions and Thoughts*

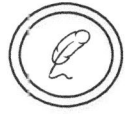

# City Roundup: Manhattan Mystiques – A Toast to Timeless Beauty and Self-Discovery

In the enchanting world of "Urban Elixir: NYC's Proven Blueprint to Timeless Skin," we've embarked on a journey through the heart of Manhattan, exploring the secrets of beauty, self-care, and the timeless allure of the city that never sleeps. From the Upper East Side's nightly rituals to Tribeca's balancing elixirs, from Brooklyn Bridge's hydration to the mysteries of the midnight hour, we've delved deep into the Manhattan mystique.

As we conclude this captivating exploration in City Roundup: Manhattan Mystiques—A Toast to Timeless Beauty and Self-Discovery, we reflect on the essence of this urban oasis. Manhattan isn't just a place; it's a state of mind. It's a city where dreams are nurtured, where beauty is an art form, and where every corner holds a story waiting to be uncovered.

In the heart of Manhattan, we've discovered that beauty is not merely skin deep; it's a reflection of one's inner self. It's about embracing the diversity of this city, finding balance amid its chaos, and surrendering to its timeless allure. It's about cherishing the moments of self-care, whether in a tranquil spa or amidst the vibrant city lights.

City Roundup: Manhattan Mystiques is a celebration of the Manhattan mystique, a reminder that beauty is a journey, not a destination. It's an ode to self-discovery, self-care, and the profound connection between inner and outer beauty. In the bustling streets of this metropolis, we've found serenity, in its towering skyscrapers, we've discovered strength, and in its diverse neighborhoods, we've uncovered the secrets to timeless skin.

So, as we bid farewell to this enchanting journey, let us carry with us the wisdom of the city, the magic of its elixirs, and the allure of its mysteries. In the pages of "Urban Elixir," Manhattan has revealed its blueprint to timeless skin, but it has also unveiled the path to unraveling our inner selves. Here's to embracing the mystique of Manhattan, and to becoming the best version of ourselves, one chapter at a time.

## Urban Elixir Recap Checklist

The Manhattan Diaries program series recap checklist—completes step five of your 21 step journey. Think of this program as a time release supplement that does its magic over the course of 21 steps, days, or weeks—you set your schedule. By committing to one chapter each morning—or one book each day or week—in 21 short days or weeks you will be able to change your life into a new You. In this book, we covered:

### 1. Manhattan Mornings: The Wake-Up Rituals for Glowing City Skin

In the opening chapter of Urban Elixir, the narrative introduces Manhattan's early morning rituals that rejuvenate the city's inhabitants, enhancing their skin with a radiant glow. This chapter delves into a luxurious skincare routine while capturing the essence of Manhattan's dawn, promising to reveal the secrets to achieving the city's signature morning radiance.

### 2. SoHo Serums: The Magic Potions Every New Yorker Swears By

In the second chapter of Urban Elixir, we delve into the allure of SoHo Serums, essential elixirs that embody Manhattan's spirit of resilience and reinvention. This narrative explores how these transformative serums enhance skin luminance and infuse users with the essence of SoHo, blending skincare with the artistry and passion of the city. It reveals the intimate connection between personal rejuvenation and the vibrant, ever-evolving urban life, urging readers to embrace reinvention as a lifestyle in Manhattan.

### 3. Met Gala Masks: Indulgent Treatments for an Event-Ready Complexion

In the third chapter of Urban Elixir, the focus shifts to achieving the Met Gala Glow, a pinnacle of Manhattan skincare luxury. This section unveils the opulent treatments and masks that prep the city's elite for the red carpet, blending timeless elegance with innovative beauty rituals. It portrays skincare as an integral part of embracing and radiating Manhattan's grandeur, setting the stage for readers to shine at the city's most glamorous events.

### 4. Central Park Cleanse: Detoxing Your Skin from City Pollutants

In the fourth chapter of Urban Elixir, we discover the Central Park Cleanse, a regimen that detoxes the skin from Manhattan's pollutants. This narrative introduces daily rituals that cleanse and rejuvenate, maintaining skin's radiance despite the city's grime. It delves into the balance of embracing city life while protecting one's glow, offering a fresh start every morning in Manhattan's relentless pace.

### 5. Broadway's Barrier Boost: Strengthening Defenses Against Urban Elements

In the fifth chapter of Urban Elixir, we explore Broadway's Barrier Boost, a skincare regimen designed to protect against Manhattan's harsh elements. This chapter reveals the protective routines that help city dwellers maintain their skin's health and radiance, even in the face of urban challenges. It emphasizes the importance of fortifying the skin with carefully selected elixirs and spritzes, allowing one to navigate the city confidently and emerge unscathed, every day poised as their own opening night.

## 6. Fifth Avenue Facials: The Elite's Go-To for Monthly Skin Refinement

In the sixth chapter of Urban Elixir, we explore the Fifth Avenue Facial, a luxurious skin care ritual favored by Manhattan's elite. This chapter delves into exclusive treatments that blend ancient techniques with modern innovation, emphasizing skin refinement as a ritual rather than a luxury. It highlights how these facials are not merely about aesthetic enhancement but are deeply intertwined with the city's vibrant pulse, allowing individuals to embody and reflect Manhattan's dynamic energy and elegance.

## 7. Tribeca Tonics: The Balancing Act for Lustrous, Even Tones

In the seventh chapter of Urban Elixir, we explore Tribeca Tonics, which are essential for achieving a balanced and lustrous skin tone. This chapter delves into the sophisticated world of skin care in Tribeca, blending age-old remedies with modern innovations to create elixirs that mirror the vibrancy of Manhattan. It highlights how these tonics not only enhance aesthetic beauty but also resonate with the city's dynamic rhythm, making each user's skin a reflection of Manhattan's diverse and vibrant character.

## 8. Brooklyn Bridge Barrier Creams: Crossing Over to Ultimate Hydration

In the eighth chapter of Urban Elixir, we delve into Brooklyn Bridge Barrier Creams, which are vital for achieving deep skin hydration. This section highlights how these creams not only provide moisture but also embody the vibrant essence of Manhattan, protecting the skin from urban stressors. The narrative connects skincare with the city's dynamic spirit, encouraging readers to embrace a routine that nourishes and reflects Manhattan's unique energy.

## 9. Upper East Side Elixirs: Nightly Rituals for Maximum Regeneration

In the ninth chapter of Urban Elixir, we explore the Upper East Side Elixirs, focusing on nightly skincare rituals that maximize skin regeneration. This chapter unveils potent potions and serums that transform and rejuvenate, syncing with Manhattan's nocturnal pace. It highlights how these rituals, more than mere skincare, offer a rebirth each morning, promising renewal and elegance that mirror the Upper East Side's refined lifestyle.

## 10. NYC Nightcap: Embracing Sleep, the Skin's Best Kept Secret

In the tenth chapter of Urban Elixir, we delve into the transformative power of sleep for maintaining radiant skin amidst Manhattan's sleepless energy. This chapter highlights essential nighttime rituals, like using silk sleep masks and lavender scents, that enhance sleep quality and promote skin rejuvenation. It emphasizes the importance of aligning with the city's quieter moments to awaken with a glow that mirrors the energy and elegance of Manhattan at dawn.

## Where Do We Go From Here?

In the vibrant tapestry of Manhattan, as we conclude our journey through the pages of "Urban Elixir: NYC's Proven Blueprint to Timeless Skin," part of the Manhattan Allure—Just Like That mini-series, we find ourselves at a crossroads, pondering the question: Where do we go from here?

In this bustling metropolis, the possibilities are endless, and the streets are paved with dreams waiting to be realized. We've embarked on a quest for timeless skin, delving into the secrets of beauty and self-care that Manhattan has graciously shared with us. We've learned that beauty is not just about aesthetics but also a reflection of our inner selves.

As we transition from one chapter to the next, let us carry the wisdom of Manhattan's elixirs with us. Let us remember that beauty is a journey of self-discovery, a path to inner and outer radiance. Beyond the skincare routines and spa rituals, there lies a world of opportunities, experiences, and adventures waiting for us.

In the upcoming pages of "Eat Like an A-Lister: Manhattan's Ultimate Nutrition Guide," part of the Manhattan Vitality—Just Like That mini-series, we will explore another facet of self-care—nourishing our bodies from the inside out. Manhattan has a lot more to offer, and it's time to embrace the vitality that this city exudes.

So, where do we go from here? We move forward with open hearts and a thirst for new experiences. We continue our journey of self-discovery, seeking not only timeless skin but also a timeless connection with the heartbeat of Manhattan. In the city that never sleeps, our adventures are just beginning, and the best is yet to come. Cheers to the next book, where we'll eat like A-listers and discover the true vitality of Manhattan.

# CITY ROUNDUP

*Completed Tasks: Recap Checklist Activities*

---

---

---

---

---

---

---

---

---

---

---

---

---

---

---

---

---

---

---

---

---

---

---

---

---

---

---

---

---

---

---

---

---

---

---

*Inspirational Quote*

LORD, GRANT THAT I MAY ALWAYS DESIRE MORE THAN I CAN ACCOMPLISH. — Michelangelo

*Action Items: Intentions and Thoughts*

# Journal Pages: Pen Your Tales

# Journal Pages: Pen Your Tales

*Journal Pages: Pen Your Tales*

*Journal Pages: Pen Your Tales*

# Journal Pages: Pen Your Tales

*Journal Pages: Pen Your Tales*

# Journal Pages: Pen Your Tales

*Journal Pages: Pen Your Tales*

*Journal Pages: Pen Your Tales*

*Journal Pages: Pen Your Tales*

www.ingramcontent.com/pod-product-compliance
Lightning Source LLC
Chambersburg PA
CBHW032054020426
42335CB00011B/330